CONDUCTIVE EDUCATION FOR ADULT HEMIPLEGIA

CONDUCTIVE EDUCATION FOR ADULT HEMIPLEGIA

ESTER COTTON MCSP

Advisory Physiotherapist to the Spastics Society, London

ROWENA KINSMAN MCSP

Superintendent Physiotherapist, Barnet General Hospital, Barnet, Hertfordshire

Churchill Livingstone 🏛

EDINBURGH LONDON MELBOURNE AND NEW YORK 1983

CHURCHILL LIVINGSTONE
Medical Division of Longman Group Limited

Distributed in the United States of America by
Churchill Livingstone Inc., 1560 Broadway, New York,
N.Y. 10036, and by associated companies, branches
and representatives throughout the world.

First published 1983

ISBN 0 443 02723 4

British Library Cataloguing in Publication Data

Cotton, Ester
   Conductive education for adult hemiplegia.
   1. Hemiplegia   2. Physical therapy
   I. Title   II. Kinsman, Rowena
   616.8'37062   RC385

Library of Congress Cataloging in Publication Data

Cotton, Ester.
   Conductive education for adult hemiplegia.

   Bibliography: p.
   1. Hemiplegics—Rehabilitation.   2. Hemiplegics—
Education.   I. Kinsman, Rowena.   II. Title.
RC406.H45C67   1983   617   82-23626

Printed in Singapore by
Huntsmen Offset Printing Ltd.

Preface

This book has been written in response to the many enquiries about our recent work in the field of Conductive Education with adult hemiplegia. It is based on Ester Cotton's observations at the Institute for the Motor Disabled in Budapest; our experiences over several years with groups at Queen Mary's Hospital, Roehampton, the Whittington Hospital, Highgate and Barnet General Hospital; last but not least, on lecture notes and task-series given by Professor Petö to Ester Cotton. The Institute for Conductive Education of the Motor Disabled and Conductor's College was founded in Budapest by Professor Petö in 1945. Since his death in 1967, it has been under the leadership of his pupil and co-operator, Dr Maria Hari. The Institute is a rehabilitation centre primarily for children, the majority of whom are residential; it is neither a hospital nor a school but is regarded as a pre-school training centre from which children move into suitable schools as soon as possible. There is a large out-patient department for babies and adult neurological conditions, who may also be treated as in-patients.

London, 1983   E.C. R.K.

Acknowledgements

Thanks are due to many people who have given help and advice with the preparation of this book. Particular assistance has been given by:

The Chest, Heart and Stroke Association, who financed translation of Professor Petö's lecture notes

Dr Maria Hari, for her continued interest in our work in Great Britain

Mrs Susan Gorka, who so ably translated the work

Dr T. Dormandy, who gave us his time, read the original lecture notes and advised on their contents

Miss Eli Kinnear, who has developed with great skill the group at Queen Mary's Hospital, Roehampton

The Association of Chartered Physiotherapists with Special Interest in Neurology

Mrs Jenny Black, Mrs Rita Milligan and Mrs Dana Telford, for their patience and assistance with the typing

Mr Francis Doddington, for providing the photographs

Miss Judith Matheson, for the illustration and design of sections of the book

Miss Anne Dummett, for her careful proof-reading

Explanatory Note

Ester Cotton

Over a decade ago I visited Professor Petö's Institute for the Motor Disabled and Conductor's College in Budapest. I never imagined on that sunny morning that I would become so interested in Conductive Education and spend so much of my time proclaiming this system.

As for hemiplegia, all I saw that morning were large groups of patients working for very long hours. At that time I was so prejudiced against group work—in favour of individual therapy—that I could hardly concentrate on the outcome of the session. But it did strike me suddenly and forcibly that after prolonged effort these patients actually lifted up their hemiplegic arms with extended elbows. I listened to the rhythmical sound of their speech but did not understand why they spoke and what influence this had on their performance. In fact, their speech had a soporific influence on me in the warm room.

I had on that day a conversation with Professor Petö. When I enquired about the speech, he only said they used the second signalling system. Later he mentioned Luria and his book. *The Role of Speech in the Regulation of Normal and Abnormal Behaviour.* When I left Budapest, after my second visit to the Institute, I was still very confused and not yet particularly interested in the work of the Institute. However, what had impressed me most were the girls who worked with the hemiplegic patients. They were so insistent and so seriously encouraging, creating a very special atmosphere in the group. This was very different from the jolly group work that I knew from England, which although pleasant, did not create the right atmosphere for learning—as for individual treatment, I was aware that patients often become too attached to their therapists. Both these factors were foreign to Conductive Education.

I intended to return again to Budapest, and therefore made enquiries in varying quarters as to the function of the patients' speech. Speech therapists I consulted had never heard of the second signalling system, and the neurologists I spoke to were not familiar with Luria's work. This was the first time in my life that I had experienced the lack of communication caused by the Iron Curtain between the East and West. In continuing my search for information, I found there were many other 'curtains', most notably those dividing the professions. It was not until I met neuropsychologists that I was able to obtain answers to my questions.

The problem of integration of the professions has shown itself as more and more difficult and the solution in the West has been to introduce the multi-disciplinary team. When I tried to introduce Conductive Education, as applied to children with cerebral palsy, I discovered how insecure the professionals were and how frightened they became if the citadels they built around themselves were threatened. Professor Petö knew this well and solved the problem by creating a new professional—the Conductor. Young girls train for four years and learn to deal with all problems facing a patient with a neurological deficit. In this way, Petö gives the patients a chance to function as a whole instead of in fragments. As fragmentation and confusion are the patient's worst enemies, the results of Conductive Education are immediate, because the patient feels secure.

Until a few years ago I was only involved in developing Conductive Education amongst children with cerebral palsy. In this I have had excellent support from the Spastics Society, especially its late Director, Mr James Loring, now Chairman of the International Cerebral Palsy Society. The Petö Unit at Ingfield Manor School, for young children suffering from cerebral palsy, is the outcome of this work.

Contents

PART ONE
The System

Introduction: background to Conductive Education
HISTORICAL BACKGROUND

Prior to the Second World War, the hemiplegic patient was often the 'Cinderella' of the Physiotherapy Department. The physiotherapist used her traditional tools of the trade—massage, passive movements, active movements, heat, cold, electrotherapy, slings, bandages, calipers. Any combination of these became recognized as 'conventional' physiotherapy. The patient was encouraged to compensate with the unaffected side; the efforts and associated reactions often increasing spasticity and leading to contractures —ultimately to the 'one-sided' individual.

As long ago as 1860 the neurologist John Hughling-Jackson hypothesized that areas of the motor cortex represented muscles on the opposite side of the body. Nearly fifty years went by before other neurologists and physiologists began to map out areas of the brain, propose channels of communication (Sir Charles Sherrington, 1934 to 1942) and the analysis of function of movement (Bernstein 1935). As theories became more widely known it was not surprising that pioneers in the field of physiotherapy began to acquaint themselves with these advances and develop neurophysiological approaches to the treatment of hemiplegia. 'Conventional' physiotherapy may still be used, but most physiotherapists are now aware of more specific approaches to the treatment of adult hemiplegia. Most notable in this field are Dr and Mrs Bobath, Dr Kabat, Miss Rood, Dr Twitchell, Miss Brunstrom and Dr Temple Fay. Each of these pioneers used neurophysiological approaches to enable the therapist to tackle the problems of the neurological deficits. While differing in emphasis, techniques and facilitations, there are some features common to them all:

1. The theoretical background is western neuro-physiology

2. Treatment is directed towards the affected side to:

    reduce spasticity (hypertonia)

    improve sensory input and propricoceptive feedback

    reduce reflex activity or use reflex activity

    break up stereotyped motor patterns

    facilitate normal movement

3. Treatment is divided between physio-therapy, occupational therapy and speech therapy

4. Treatment sessions are by appointment and have little connection with the rhythm of the day-to-day routine

5. The outcome of treatment is in the hands of the therapists, who use a variety of techniques—for example, handling, positioning, pressure, manual facilitations, icing, brushing, tapping

6. Treatment of the patient is often isolated from the management of the patient, with areas of overlap not developed to full potential, allowing for poor reinforcement and a lack of continuity

THE DEVELOPMENT OF PROFESSOR PETÖ'S SYSTEM—CONDUCTIVE EDUCATION

Professor Petö, in common with the others in this field, wanted to break up motor patterns, reduce spasticity and develop more selective movements. However, unlike his contemporaries, Professor Petö chose to rely on *the patient's own active participation and initiative* rather than on the handling and skill of the therapist. With this aim he moved into the educational and neuropsychological field where he was inspired by the works of Pavlov, Luria, Vygotsky, Bernstein and others. This step into the world of *education* enabled Professor Petö to develop his new and original approach to the rehabilitation of neurological conditions.

Therapists who wish to interest themselves in Conductive Education will not only have to acquire the techniques of this system but must also widen their theoretical knowledge to include learning theories and information about voluntary movements (the motor act), and study how skills are acquired.

The Russian physiologist Pavlov, in his famous experiments, showed that dogs could be conditioned to associate stimuli with reward. This represented a simple form of learning, which became known as *classical conditioning*, or *learning by association*. Normally dogs salivate when presented with food. This involuntary response Pavlov called the *unconditional response* (UCR) and the stimulus he called the *unconditioned stimulus* (UCS).

Food ⟶ salivation

(UCS)   (UCR)

He noted that if some other stimulus (e.g. sound or light) accompanied or preceded the food, it evoked the same response. This stimulus he called the *conditioned stimulus* (CS). This second stimulus on its own did not evoke a response, but in association with the unconditioned stimulus, i.e. food, it did.

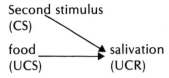

Second stimulus
(CS)

food   salivation
(UCS)   (UCR)

The association between a conditioned stimulus and a *conditioned response* is learned through the pairing of these two stimuli followed by the unconditioned response. After repeated presentation of the conditioned stimulus it would itself become enough to elicit salivation. In other words salivation occurred independently of the unconditioned stimulus.

conditioned stimulus ⟶ conditioned response

However, it was found necessary to re-introduce the unconditioned stimulus to strengthen the link between the UCS and CS. This Pavlov called *reinforcement*. If the conditioned stimulus is repeatedly presented without the accompaniment of the UCS then the conditioned response ceases to occur. This is known as *extinction*.

Once a conditioned response is linked to a conditioned stimulus, other similar stimuli will evoke the same response. This is known as *generalization* and accounts for our being able to react to new situations in so far as they resemble familiar ones.

As Pavlov extended his experiments he developed elaborate chains of conditioned stimuli. He noted that with dogs the more complex the chain the less the success rate was; this was not so with human beings. He argued that this was because language used as conditioned stimuli is a strong reinforcer. He called this conditioned stimulus, i.e. language, 'the second signalling system, peculiarly ours, the signal of signals which has made us human'.

All hemiplegic patients have to relearn voluntary movements. The origins of voluntary movement (the motor act) have been studied as far back as Descartes and still remains largely a mystery. Two schools of thought dominate—the *idealistic* and the *mechanistic*. The former suggests that a voluntary movement arises from an act of will which evokes a movement. The latter rests on the idea that voluntary movements are only responses to external stimuli (Setchenov), an approach that proved applicable only to very simple programmes.

Bernstein maintained that the human motor act is so varied that the mechanistic approach was insufficient. Vygotsky took this argument further by suggesting that the basis of voluntary movement in childhood is social in origin and arises in communication between adult and child. In early years a child's behaviour is regulated by adult speech, i.e. 'give me, take it' etc. Later, when he has learned to speak and can give himself spoken instructions, he will begin to influence his own development and behaviour. Acquisition of skills is sequential, varying with age and ability. In the early stages of maturation a child learns by trial and error; his efforts are assisted by his mother, who will guide and improve his performance both manually and verbally. During this period the child depends on the progress of his physical development to make the skill possible; for instance, a child of 6 months can pull off his sock because he can stabilize his trunk, bend his hips and grasp his foot, while also co-ordinating hand and eye for the task. As already mentioned, this skill is achieved through trial and error. At later stages of learning the mother will use a great deal of language which will also help the child's cognitive learning—e.g. in the task of putting on a vest, where the mother gives step-by-step instruction. The more complicated the task the more precise will be the language. A useful analogy in adult life is the experience of learning to drive a car, where the instructor guides the learner solely through verbal instruction and gradually 'internal speech' becomes the regulator of the skill.

In his book *The Role of Speech in the Regulation of Normal and Abnormal Behaviour*, Luria explored the reinforcing influence of speech on motor behaviour. As movements are learnt they can be carried out without accompanied speech or by repeating words silently (internal speech). The intention is constant and represents a future need, the goal also being constant. The road to the goal moves through many stages (referred to by Connolly as *sub-goals*, *task-parts* or *sub-routes*). An active movement starts with an intention and finishes with a goal, and it is not the movement but the goal which is represented in the motor cortex. Luria further hypothesized that brain-damaged people whose selection process is impaired could be retained to select required information, essential for being able to tackle everyday tasks. It has to be remembered that any motor act involves constant monitoring between the action or actions performed and the original intention. For the original intention to be performed successfully this analysis and comparison is absolutely vital.

In Conductive Education the patient learns a task which will lead to the acquisition of skills. Initially he attempts the whole task observed by the Conductor. The task is then broken up into appropriate task-parts. As the task parts are mastered, these intermediate steps are assimilated and new task-parts are introduced. In this way the patient develops a wider repertoire of movement. Unless the various combinations are learnt, the patient will fail in his attempts to perform the task in a controlled way. The patient is taught how to guide his movements towards each task-part of the task by using his own speech (*Rhythmical Intention*).

Further to fully understanding Professor

Petö's approach to treatment compared with his contemporaries, it is essential to understand his concept of dysfunction versus orthofunction. He rejected the narrow view of dysfunction as mere motor disability (i.e. handicap) and maintained that dysfunctions are partial manifestations of a neurological disorder which arise from a breakdown of general adaptive development and affect the entire personality.

Function is bound up with the successful performance of tasks that arise from the biological and social system of demands appropriate to a particular stage of life. It should be remembered that with increasing age there is less hope of spontaneous adaptation. Therefore to achieve recovery there is need for expert guidance (*Conduction*). It is by considering the relationship between the individual and his environment that a full understanding of dysfunction is possible. Cerebral dysfunction results in changes of the personality and ability to adapt, which govern the patient's learning ability. The word 'learning' should be taken in its widest sense and includes every aspect of the patient's personality. Education and adaptation are concerned with the problems of *learning*, therefore the rehabilitation of patients with dysfunction is an *educational task*.

In conclusion, the system of Conductive Education is concerned with teaching 'dysfunctional' persons to become functional by developing their adaptive and learning abilities. Conductive Education is a totally integrated system, and the operator of the system is the *Conductor*.

The role of the Conductor

Professor Petö, by his definition of dysfunction, created a need for a new professional, namely, the Conductor. The Conductor* is the person who co-ordinates the patient's day so that he may perform to his best ability intellectually, emotionally and physically.

The Institute in Budapest, besides being a treatment centre, is a training college for Conductors; the training takes four years. Conductors are mainly female and are accepted on A-level equivalent qualifications. They must also show an aptitude for the work. The Hungarian Ministry of Education recognises the professional qualification awarded to Conductors graduating from the Institute.

The syllabus is demanding and includes anatomy, physiology, neurology, pathology, paediatrics, psychology, nursery skills, nursery teacher and infant teacher subjects, movement theories, group dynamics, treatment methods and techniques, splint making and workshop routines. The student Conductor is expected to work in the Institute for six hours a day, as well as to attend lectures and complete homework. The theory taught in the lectures is put into practice at once, thereby providing immediate reinforcement.

As with others involved in caring and rehabilitation, it is important that the Conductor develops a singular personality — positive and dynamic and, wherever possible, musical.

The following are the Conductor's responsibilities:

1. a) To assess each patient
   b) To observe each patient in normal life situations
   c) To observe the patient in a group situation

*Throughout this book the Conductor is referred to as 'she' and the patient as 'he'. This is purely for the authors' convenience.

These observations and assessment form the basis on which the Conductor decides which group the patient will be allocated to.

2. *To organise and direct the timetable and day routine*

The Conductor must have contact with the patients in the broadest sense of the word, to ensure that what the patient learns in one situation is used correctly during the day, for example, when eating, drinking, washing, toileting and walking. She also plays an active part in assisting the patients to arrange their leisure time (pp. 6 & 20).

3. *To initiate the patients into the group*

All activities are programmed for the same time every day so that a work rhythm is established which helps the patient to adjust to the new way of life. The Conductor makes sure that each patient is fully aware of the timetable and that the patient becomes conditioned to this rhythm and feels secure. Activities which previously might have caused apprehension are now accepted and confusion is eliminated.

4. *To direct the group*

The Conductor can be compared with the conductor of an orchestra. She assures the smooth flow of the timetable and the repetition of harmonious movements. The patients are brought together 'in tune' through the Conductor's pleasant manner and ability to facilitate the group.

5. *To make up the task-series*

The task-series consist of many combinations of task-parts which together lead to the performance of more complicated tasks. They are not exercises.

The Conductor not only works out the task-series but is also responsible for the discarding of task-parts when they become superfluous.

6. *To create a pleasant working atmosphere*

The Conductor is responsible for arranging the room and the furniture for the patients, so that patients know they are expected and welcome.

THE ROLE OF THE FIRST AND SECOND CONDUCTORS

Two Conductors work with each group (three if the group is very large). All Conductors have the same training and are equally knowledgeable about the patients, the timetable and the task-series.

The first Conductor leads the group and initiates Rhythmical Intention (ri). She decides if a task-part has to be repeated or changed.

The second Conductor is there to assist the patients, which she does by moving from patient to patient anticipating their needs. She also helps in Rhythmical Intention and, if further repetition is needed, signals to the first Conductor accordingly. When necessary, she may use facilitations.

The Conductors may change roles during the day.

Although we recognise that in Britain there are at present no training courses for Conductors, it has been found that through staff meetings, case conferences, daily group discussions and combined efforts in making up programmes, certain individuals take up the role of 'conductor'. The authors believe that, provided the multi-disciplinary team is prepared to adopt the Conductor principle, it is possible to train any members of the team to become Conductors. This demands a dedicated staff who are versatile, willing to work shift hours and prepared to share their professional expertise.

The structure of groups

In Conductive Education, group work is the accepted format of work sessions. Patients work together in homogeneous groups which stimulate, motivate and develop their initiative. The groups are led by a Conductor who has previously planned the sessions and subsequent functional tasks. In the group setting she observes the general attitude and bearing of each patient in addition to his performance and disposition.

Besides obtaining a total view, each patient is observed individually (p. 8). Using this information, the Conductor is able to select the right group for each patient. The advantages of group work are many and varied — patients often have feelings of isolation, rejection and loneliness culminating in difficulties in forming personal relationships.

In the group the patients work together and identify with each other, sharing individual problems during rest and free periods. They find that their feelings are accepted, trust begins to develop and through this interaction confidence and their own personalities develop.

With the aid of Rhythmical Intention, and through the Conductor, the patient learns tasks (or task-parts) and how to carry these over into the rest of the day. The patients' arousal level is maintained without fatigue by working in rhythmical sequence and at a slow tempo for long periods of time.

The patient is free to choose whether he works or not. This choice allows him to develop his own self-esteem and his social awareness. The patient may also learn by watching the performance of others (vicarious learning).

Group work may take place

— at the table
— in supine lying
— in free sitting
— in standing
— in walking

It is important that at all times each patient has sufficient space so that movement is not hampered. For example, in *Task-series sitting at a table* (p. 28) patients should face each other across the table with enough space for them to extend the arms freely in all directions.

In summary, the advantages of group work are

1. motivation
2. development of initiative
3. learning of motor skills
4. vicarious learning
5. stimulation
6. social interaction

In addition to these above-mentioned advantages, the Conductor alone has continual interaction with each person, which gives her a unique opportunity of enhancing the habilitation of each patient.

SELECTION OF PATIENTS FOR GROUPS

Initially, the Conductor uses a task-series to observe the patient's ability within the group and completes an assessment of each individual patient. Using this information the patient is allocated to the most suitable group. However, it is not always possible to place a patient in the right group, so the following comments may serve as a guide line.

1. Beginners group

This group includes patients who are not ambulant and those unable to initiate voluntary movements with their affected arm. There may also be other associated problems: hemianopia, proprioceptive loss, aphasia and severe spasticity or flaccidity. The beginners group carries out task-series in lying (sometimes also in sitting). The goal of this group is to learn to raise the affected arm from the shoulder, with an extended elbow, and to place the fingers above their head. The task-series will always include grosser and finer hand movements.

In this group patients will develop body-image and spatial awareness so that without help and without Rhythmical Intention they will be able to find their own starting positions — head in the middle, arms at the side and legs straight. They also learn how to break up the total motor pattern. Patients remain in this group until such time as they can raise the affected arm from the shoulder with their elbow extended and are able to place their fingers above their head.

2. Intermediate group

Patients in this group should be able to place their clasped hands on the table whilst sitting. Patients do many task-series at the table both sitting and standing, developing hand function with extension of the elbows. Initially, they learn how to work with both hands together, moving on to positions in which one hand supports whilst the other hand moves. The patients are continually encouraged to reinforce their actions through visual feedback.

Standing up and sitting down at the table using both hands for weight-bearing through extended elbows, as well as weight transfers, are tasks included in this group in preparation for walking.

3. Advanced group

The ultimate aim for the members of the advanced group is to achieve functional independence, including free walking as well as fine movements of the affected hand.

Patients in this group may be at many different levels and therefore for some tasks may be divided into sub-groups.

It should be emphasised that this is the most difficult group to conduct because of the many different levels of individual achievement and personal expectations. Both Conductor and patient must be aware of the individual aim for the patient, and the patient should learn to identify his needs within the task-series. There is a continual interaction between the Conductor and the patient — the dynamic expectancy of the Conductor motivating the patient to achieve optimal function.

The aphasic group

It is a misconception to believe that the aphasic patient cannot be helped through Conductive Education, above all through Rhythmical Intention. It is often thought that learning a motor act through language would be an impossibility for aphasic patients: they need, in particular, specialised help to deal with the language problems. However, there are many factors other than language in Conductive Education that may facilitate comprehending and learning functional tasks for the patient — the group, observation of other patients, auditory input combined with the motor act, and the intention of the action.

All these factors, together with repetition and reinforcement, help the patient to achieve function. These patients, as in other groups, must be free to choose to work or not. They may often join in with the counting or in the dynamic commands of the task-parts when they do participate in the group.

Observation of the patient

It is worth recalling that during normal movement the central nervous system is fed precise information regarding muscle activity. Immediately any altered demand is detected, compensatory adjustments are made to result in a smooth movement. The body is programming an effective performance. This programming is part of a finely-balanced system. The hemiplegic patient with abnormal muscle behaviour is unable to programme his performance in this way.

Meticulous observation of each patient will indicate where abnormalities are and also build up a comprehensive understanding of the patient's attitude toward commands, his sense of effort and how he is able to integrate information. Observation must begin at once and continue throughout the patient's course of treatment.

In Conductive Education observation is concerned with the execution of movement that can be used for functional tasks. How each task is performed shows the Conductor where the difficulties are so that the patient can be taught how to programme his performance.

Observation of movement is divided into seven parts. These parts are not chosen arbitrarily but show how a patient performs a movement, whether he

— understands the task
— has correct body-image
— has spatial awareness

Flat hands on the stomach is chosen because it illustrates particularly well how the patient deals with his loss of ability, and encompasses the three areas mentioned above. Each therefore gives an indication of the patient's functional level. Movements are observed in supine lying, in sitting and in standing.

It is also important to be aware of the patient's attitude; for example, does he

— become angry when trying to exert himself?
— perform unnecessary movements?
— try to use the affected arm?
— prefer the unaffected arm or give up altogether?

Observation of movement	Supine Lying		Sitting		Standing	
	Yes	No	Yes	No	Yes	No

1. *Flat hands on the stomach.* Starting position:
   hands at the side. Can the patient

   — place affected hand on stomach?

   and then, can the patient

   — make a fist?

   — release fist?

   — slide hand on to chest?

   — take hand to neck?

   — take hand to back of neck?

   — take hand to opposite shoulder?

   — take hand to opposite elbow?

Comments

2. *Clasping of the hands.* Starting position: hands at the side
   Can the patient

   — clasp hands together?

   — raise clasped hands with straight elbows?

   — raise arms to 180°?

   — turn hands 'inside out'?

   — place hands (clasped) behind neck?

   — with clasped hands, touch alternate ears?

Comments

	Supine Lying		Sitting		Standing	
	Yes	No	Yes	No	Yes	No

3. *Movement of the affected arm.* Starting position: hands by sides.
Can the patient

— lift his arm with straight elbow?

— hold the extended position?

— bend his elbow?

— place the heel of his hand upon his forehead?

— place his hand on surface and push down?

— approximate finger pads of both hands ('make a basket')?

— move his thumbs individually?

— move his index finger individually?

— move his other fingers individually?

If not, can he move affected arm when above his head?

Comments

	Sitting	
	Yes	No

4. *Sitting.* Starting position: sitting with arms by sides.
Can the patient

— place hands with abducted thumbs on knees?

_____ _____

— place hand on a chair rung or table?

_____ _____

If not can he

— place hand on chair rung (with clasped hands)?

_____ _____

— grip chair rung or table or make a fist?

_____ _____

— release chair rung, table or fist?

_____ _____

Comments

---

5. *Leg movements.* Starting position: sitting with arms by sides;
a chair placed in front.
Can the patient

	Sitting	
	Yes	No

— put affected leg on to chair rung?

_____ _____

— slide affected leg down side of chair?

_____ _____

	Supine Lying	
	Yes	No

Starting position: supine lying. Can the patient

— place foot flat on the mat (knee pointing up)?

_____ _____

— part legs?

_____ _____

— place affected heel on the other knee and maintain the
position?

_____ _____

— from that position, extend leg slowly?

_____ _____

Comments

	Standing	
	Yes	No

6. *Standing up.* Can the patient stand

— up by himself?

— holding on to a chair rung? _____ _____

— supporting himself with palms on table? _____ _____

— taking equal weight on his feet? _____ _____

Whilst standing are the fingers of his affected side flexed? _____ _____

Can he place his supinated palm on his buttock? _____ _____

_____ _____

Comments

7. *Walking.* Can the patient walk

— pushing a chair with two hands?

— holding a stick in both hands? _____ _____

— holding a stick in one hand? _____ _____

— with clasped hands and extended elbows? _____ _____

— can the patient swing his arms when walking? _____ _____

_____ _____

Comments

Those patients who have no difficulty with the hand movements should be observed performing more complex tasks that are directly related with function or are functional.

	Sitting	
	Yes	No

Complex hand tasks for the advanced patient. Starting position: sitting with hands by the side. Can the patient

— alternately make a fist and release it?

— bend and straighten individual fingers?

— place palm on table and individually extend his fingers?

— flick individual fingers?

— circle individual fingers?

— oppose individual fingers?

— carry a tray with both hands?

— lift a book and put if down?

— hold a book open with fingers and thumb extended?

— hold a pencil with a tripod grasp (pencil should be held vertically or horizontally)?

— let go of the pencil?

— pick pencil up again?

— take a handkerchief to his nose?

— undo a button?

— do up a button?

— tie a knot

— use a threaded needle

— thread a large-eyed needle?

— comb his hair?

Comments

Facilitations

Conductive Education is a system of learning in which everything is designed to facilitate learning. Learning requires not only a learning method but also possibilities for motivation, continuity, repetition and reinforcement. An educator who can combine all the aspects of learning in an atmosphere conducive to learning is practising Conductive Education. The word 'facilitate' means 'to make easier' and to make function easier is the aim of all those working with the hemiplegic patient. The whole system of Conductive Education acts as a facilitation. Each part—Rhythmical Intention, the timetable, individual programmes, the group, the Conductor—is as important as the others and each should be regarded as a facilitatory factor. For instance, anticipation of success is created by the Conductor, who expects and welcomes her patients and is ready to start each day punctually. The timing of the day's programme is such that the patient can move effortlessly from one task to another. The aim of the programme is to overcome both inertia and apathy and to help the patient develop a feeling of achievement.

In Conductive Education there are individual facilitations that should be clearly understood and then integrated into the programme by the Conductor. These are

1. Rhythmical Intention
2. Motivation
3. Continuity
4. Self-facilitations
5. Manual facilitations

Facilitations may be regarded as supports, or that which is required for the successful completion of the task. As the patient improves, these supports are removed.

1. RHYTHMICAL INTENTION

Rhythmical Intention (ri) is the correct wording of each task-part (p. 19), first spoken by the Conductor and then repeated by the Conductor and the group *before* any movement takes place. The movement is carried out following the intention, using counting or dynamic speech. The correct wording is important, as these words build up the patient's understanding of movement, body-image and spatial awareness. The counting should be neither too fast nor too slow and the Conductor should allow the patients to use internal speech (see p. 3).

The hemiplegic patient no longer has the easy ability to formulate motor plans: e.g., picking up an object is always done in the familiar pattern of elbow flexion, pronation and flexion of the wrist and flexion of the hand. In Conductive Education, Rhythmical Intention is used to teach the patient *actively* how to break up these stereotyped patterns and plan more selective movements by the use of language. The patient learns how to perform a movement, and it is the careful structure of the task-parts combined with Rhythmical Intention that develops the patient's understanding of the motor plan as well as his motor memory. Rhythmical Intention and every movement, therefore, become completely inseparable and provide a basis for a structure of such an order that it is possible to recall and reconstruct movement in the course of everyday situations. In other words, the solution of the task takes on a wider meaning until it is a way of life and the patient is able to execute movements without verbal facilitations.

So that movement is possible, the hemiplegic patient must learn to control his own spasticity. Initially he prepares himself for a task by deliberately inhibiting spasticity (loosening up) with the use of Rhythmical Intention, correct starting position and gravity, e.g. 'my hands are hanging down' (1–5) (see Task-series). This preparation encourages him to perform active movements within a given time limit and with less effort. The planning of the task and the counting provide the division of time that is needed for the execution of the task. Counting is only used when prescribed and is only necessary when learning the task. Once the task is learnt and there is a wholeness of movement counting may be discarded.

If a patient cannot carry out the intention, the Conductor should ensure that the verbal instructions are such that the patient fully understands the task. It is not uncommon in hemiplegic patients to find that patients have lost the idea of movement as expressed in words, e.g. 'stretching the elbows' may be meaningless whilst 'pushing the hands forward' may be more comprehensible. In this instance the intentions may be changed, so that 'I push my hands forward' becomes 'I push my hands forward and stretch my elbows', which then can become 'I stretch my elbows'.

In this way, the patient learns not only the physical aspect of the task but begins to redevelop his understanding of movement. The rhythm, the comprehension and the self-direction all together facilitate the patient's ability to concentrate.

To sum up, Rhythmical Intention helps the patient to

1. Work for very long periods during the day
2. Produce sounds and speak while moving
3. Learn new motor patterns by establishing contact between the higher centres of the brain, the trunk and limbs
4. Develop body-image and an idea of position in space
5. Further concentration
6. Work *actively*, developing motor memory
7. Teach himself to control his own spasticity

2. MOTIVATION

Motivation is *intrinsic* and not *extrinsic*. That is, the motivation comes from the patient. The patient participates in the programme and is motivated to achieve to the maximum through his own efforts. The right task is a motivating factor. If the Conductor sets the wrong task, too difficult a task, or one that is impossible to carry out—such as early arm-raising—the patient will be discouraged by the demands made upon him.

Besides the right task motivation, Conductive Education is concerned with all the factors that energize behaviour and give it direction. Patients working in a group situation also learn through observing the others in the group. That is, patients watch each other and observe the outcome, noting that some patients are reaching goals as yet unattainable to themselves. They are then motivated by the others' successes to try harder. In effect they are modelling their actions upon those of their neighbours. The importance of body language (e.g. glancing) should not be overlooked, for it is these early glances and other movements that motivate the patient to develop a comradeship with other members. They begin to feel they belong and are motivated to interact with other group members, redeveloping lost social skills.

The Conductor should be sympathetic to the patients' emotions, recognizing that these are closely intertwined with motivation. For example, pleasure and joy are often experienced when a task is successfully completed, whereas the unsuccessful goal may bring about frustration, anger and depression—emotional feelings that tend to inhibit motivation.

3. CONTINUITY

The Conductor is the Director of the timetable. The execution of this must be an interesting experience for both the Conductor and the patient, allowing sufficient time for trial, experimentation and success. It also reinforces the learning of functional tasks in a realistic manner. The patient learns each daily-living task in the time and place required for normal functioning. The routine of the day, therefore, becomes worthwhile and proceeds without interruptions, the patient becoming conditioned to rhythm; and those activities that might previously have been the cause of apprehension or even unwillingness fall into the daily rhythm. The success of any task-series depends upon the rhythm of the day, which in turn is dependent upon the punctuality and the regular attendance of the members of the group and the Conductor. It is also the Conductor's responsibility to see that the patients carry out all day-to-day tasks correctly in their widest sense, e.g. at meal times, when attending to their personal needs or when moving around. The patient must perform all these activities with as much care as the task-parts in the task-series. The discipline of behaviour enables the patient to learn ways of achieving aims, however small these aims may be.

Every patient's time-table should include free time. The suitable use of his free time will naturally depend upon the stimulation that is provided. In the beginning this is carefully monitored as patients must learn to use time actively. Gradually, as the patients are motivated, this free time fits easily into daily rhythm.

For the purpose of explanation a useful analogy can be made with the Conductor of an orchestra. The Conductor leads the orchestra— likewise the Conductor in Conductive Education assures the smooth flow of the day's timetable and the repetition of harmonious movement. The Conductor knows all the members of his group/orchestra and their separate abilities, bringing them together/in tune. When listening to a musical composition, pleasure is derived from the recognition of certain movements. In the same way, patients taking part in an entire day's timetable/programme derive pleasure from known movements as if it were a composition.

4. SELF-FACILITATION

Hemiplegic patients can be involved in their own facilitations. That is, once a task is understood and a movement attempted, the patient can facilitate with

- vision
- pressure (using his body, furniture or other props)
- gravity
- correct starting positions
- clasping of hands
- language

The patient is encouraged to follow the direction of movements with his eyes, thereby using visual facilitation (*vision*). In this way, the task becomes more meaningful and the patient recognises the movement. If a patient experiences difficulty with clasping hands, he may be able to achieve this by firmly pressing the backs of his elbows against the inside of his knees. In this case it is the firm *pressure* of the elbows against the knees which facilitates extension of the elbow and loosening of the hand. In the final stages of rehabilitation the patient learns to separate the fingers in parting of the hands (code Y p. 25) by pressing the thumbs out. Besides using the patient's own body, it is possible to use furniture to facilitate a movement, e.g. using the edge of a table to maintain thumb abduction and extension whilst parting the hands (Task 5 Code k4 p. 37). The use of laddered chairs, benches or stools may be considered necessary equipment to teach the patient to help himself, e.g. in *Task-series in free sitting* (p. 53) the patient may use the rungs of the chair to maintain the position of the extended arm.

The Conductor, who must be aware of this, may help the patient by incorporating the effect of *gravity* into the task-part (Fig. 1), thereby inhibiting spasticity. It is essential that every patient finds his *own* starting position (which is in itself facilitatory for the task-series) and that this starting position is the correct one. The patient may use a series of positions taught to achieve the correct *starting position*, i.e. making the body in a straight line for *Task-series in supine lying.*

Clasping of the hands (Fig. 2) is an important self-facilitator. First and foremost, the patient finds satisfaction in bringing his hands together. 'It helps me feel in one piece', was one patient's expression. Professor Petö's explanation was simple—'the patient gets a grip on himself'.

Clasping of the hands also enables the patient to

- work with two hands in midline
- observe both hands
- separate the fingers
- supinate the affected hand

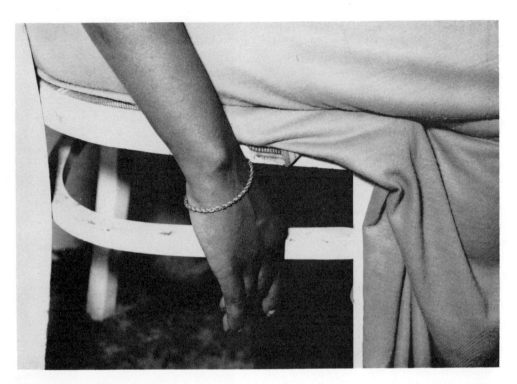

Fig. 1 Self facilitation—gravity

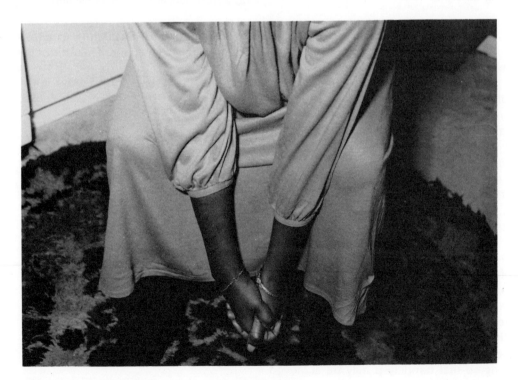

Fig. 2 Clasping of the hands using extension of the elbow

- facilitate the affected hand with the other hand
- develop extension of the elbow, wrist and fingers
- stabilize the shoulder girdle, which ultimately leads to *separation of the hands* (see codes X and Y, p. 25)

All aids and facilitations, including clasping of the hands, should be regarded as supports required for the successful completion of the task.

Language is also used as a self-facilitator. The patient learns to use Rhythmical Intention as a resource whenever he experiences difficulties with his own performance. The Conductor teaches the patient to regulate his performance by verbalising his intention prior to performing it. This will involve the Conductor in asking the patient 'What are you going to do?', instead of telling him what to do. The patient trying to stand up may say 'I lean forward, I stretch my arms, I stand up.' In this way he regulates his performance and develops a habit, with ri becoming an aid or tool.

5. MANUAL FACILITATIONS

Manual facilitations in Conductive Education are considered a last resort and are used only when all other facilitations have been tried and failed.

Manual facilitations may be performed by the first or second Conductor, or on occasion by the patient himself. Almost all facilitations are done distally, with minimal help. The Conductor may assist the patient by *fixation* (of wrist, finger, elbow or the other limb), thus enabling the patient to do the movement actively. However, if this facilitation is used repeatedly, it must be recognised that the patient is not learning. Using the example 'clasping of hands' a patient experiencing difficulty may find that this action is facilitated if the middle finger is temporarily hyper-extended. This allows for sufficient loosening so that handclasp may be achieved. Similarly, the thumb may be abducted and

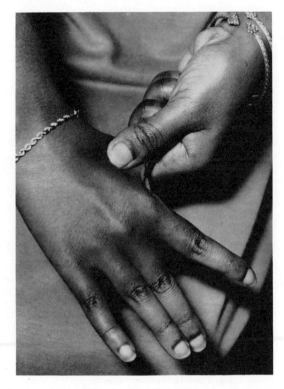

Fig. 3 Facilitation of extension of the finger

internally rotated, facilitating extension of the fingers (Fig. 3). The patient may himself manually facilitate one of the fingers if he finds this helpful.

Task-series and acquisition of skills

Conductive Education is based on the neuro-psychological theories of skill acquisition. Basic skills of manipulation and locomotion are learnt in the first two years of life. If these skills are lost, as in hemiplegia, they must be re-taught and re-learnt.

The patient is guided towards a skill by the Conductor, is motivated by the group and learns with the use of language. The patient never does exercises but works through task-series that are built up from task-parts and lead to a goal (the achieved skill).

The success of the patient depends on the Conductor's ability to choose the right task. The task must be understood by the patient and at the same time be neither too difficult nor too easy. Initially the whole task is attempted, and learning it embodies a constant movement between that whole task and the many task-parts that lead to the goal.

Assessment of the entire group from every aspect is essential before the Conductor starts work. She can then decide on the appropriate skills to be acquired and the tasks to be taught. Task-series should never be copied, but should be created according to the composition of the group. As the patients improve, new goals are set.

When planning the task-series, the Conductor must always be aware of sensory disturbances. Sometimes, with his eyes closed, the hemiplegic patient may not be able to tell whether his elbow is straight or bent, whether his palms are facing up or down. He may not know the feeling of elbow or finger-stretching and, even if he were to succeed in stretching, would not connect the movement with the idea and would therefore be unable to repeat the action. Stretching is often achieved by manual facilitation; however the patient does not always connect that with the idea of stretching.

Proprioception and perception must be supported by visual and auditory stimulation. It is for this reason that all tasks are performed with Rhythmical Intention. A kinaesthetic effect is achieved through the use of speech as a secondary sensory reinforcement.

RHYTHMICAL INTENTION

The tasks and task-parts are taught by the use of language: Rhythmical Intention. This consists of two parts, the intention and the rhythmical counting (or dynamic speech). Both must be used slowly, loudly and clearly so that the room becomes filled with sound.

The intention

Learning a skill is intentional—it starts with an intention and ends with a goal. The hemiplegic patient may experience difficulties in comprehending the intention, if this refers to his lost movements or body-awareness, and may therefore not achieve the goal. The Conductor should be aware of these difficulties and change the intentions appropriately. For example, in *Task-series sitting at a table* (p. 29) the intention 'I stretch my elbows' may produce no results; the intention 'I push my hands forwards' may result in straight elbows although the patient may be slumped on the table; however, the intention

Hands on table   (1–5)
Elbows off the table   (1–5)
Elbows on the table   (1–5)

will result in the patient sitting up whilst performing a stretching and bending of the elbows. The Conductor should then stress that the elbows are straight, so that the patients learn the intention 'I stretch my elbows'.

Rhythmical counting (or dynamic speech)

The Conductor says the intention first: 'I stretch my elbows'. This is repeated by the group and the Conductor. Only while the group and the Conductor count is the task attempted. Counting is used to give the correct timing and rhythm for the task. The Conductor may count 1–5, with the intention 'I stretch my elbows'. In this instance the counting is unemphasised. On the other hand, she may count 1,2,3,4,5 with the intention 'to make a basket', where each numeral is emphasised, thereby stressing the individual movements required (see page 34). In the same way, the Conductor may count 1–2 as when moving a foot for a step, or 1 with the intention 'I put my foot to the left' and 2 'I put my foot back'.

If the patient needs a more direct or emphatic approach, dynamic speech is used—for example, 'stretch, stretch, stretch'.

The tasks and task-series given in this book should only be regarded as examples. They have been chosen because they are essential to all hemiplegic patients. We have selected 'sitting at a table' as the first task-series. In this position patients learn to maintain the sitting position and perform task-parts using visual feedback, observing their own performance and that of the group. The second task-series is performed in lying. Initially the task-series in lying may seem easier because of the fixation of the trunk; however, they are complicated as the patient has difficulty combining arm and leg movements. He is unable easily to observe his own performance or that of others. The rest of the task-series chosen follow natural progressions—free sitting, standing and walking.

Each task-series is divided into task-parts. In front of each task-part is a letter. This letter is part of a code. The use of a code becomes apparent as the conductor develops and builds up new task-series, using it to express the task-parts accurately. It should be noted that certain combinations are used frequently. This is deliberate as these combinations emphasize learning through repetition and reinforcement. They are expressed as X, Y, Z.

X — putting two clasped hands on the table
Y — two parted, flat hands
Z — a basket

The patient should learn to memorize the sequences that go to make up these combinations (see pp. 25–26).

The conductor organizes the sequences of task-series according to the patient's or group's ability.

The full benefit of Conductive Education lies in the successful transfer of skills from one situation to another. For example, successful stretching of the fingers should not be viewed as the goal in itself unless it is used to perform a functional task.

The Conductor should ensure that there is ample opportunity during the day for the patient to repeat, reinforce and transfer newly-acquired skills. This opportunity for transfer of skills provides the reinforcement needed for learning. For example, the patient who has learnt to extend and abduct his thumb might be able to use this skill for the following functions:

— pushing down his bedclothes
— pushing down his pants
— pushing off his shoes
— grasping the edge of a table
— holding a tool
— shuffling cards

The role of Conductor in task-series is to establish the continuity of learning and achievement of functional tasks through which Conductive Education stands or falls.

THE TIMETABLE

Continuity can be established by structuring the patient's day through the use of a timetable. In this way the patient develops a daily rhythm. This will vary depending upon whether the patient is residential or not. The patient will learn to regulate performance with the timetable, for example, if breakfast is at 8.30 am he will learn to allow sufficient time to get ready for that meal. Obviously with a diurnal timetable there is room for flexibility dependent upon individual requirements. This should also take into account the fact that patients are continuously learning.

In order to benefit fully from Conductive Education, opportunities to make choices, develop potential and become aware of surroundings must be given. The timetable should therefore be all-encompassing; however, even when particular care in planning the

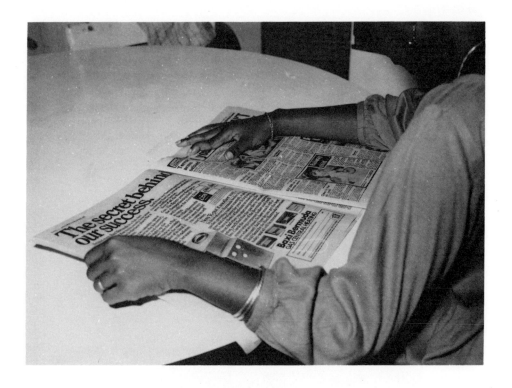

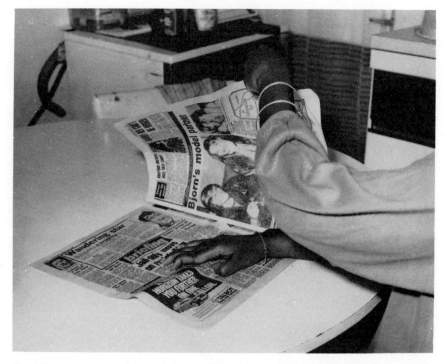

Fig. 4 Free time: using the newly learnt skills while reading a paper

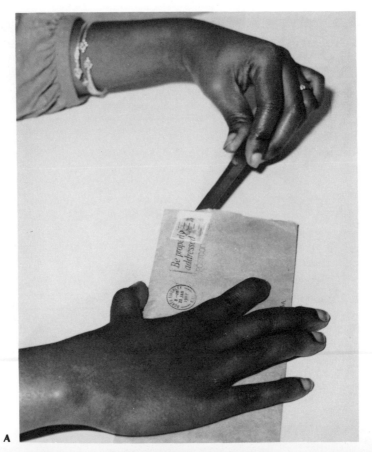

A

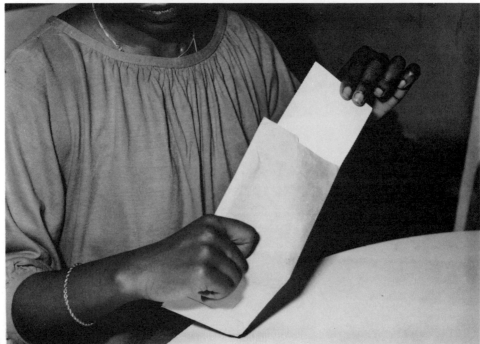

B

Fig. 5 Transfer of skills A. Opening an envelope B. Removing a letter from an envelope

day is taken, free time for the patient will inevitably occur. This can be described as *active free time*, during which the patient *actively* pursues something of his own choice, e.g. reading a newspaper (Fig. 4), or *inactive free time*. The latter occurs when nothing is happening, e.g. the patient is sitting waiting for transport.

Many of the activities incorporated into the timetable were automatic to the individual before disability occurred, but now need to be relearnt. The patient, for example, relearns to use both hands for washing and experiences again pleasure from the familiar feel of the face-cloth. At times the patient may not be able to complete a whole task—e.g. dressing—and is able only to put his arms through the sleeves of his jumper. The Conductor must be aware of this and prevent the patient from waiting in this inactive position by stepping in to help. The patient is thus aware of available help and instead of becoming frustrated with the task is daily motivated to try a bit further.

The beginning of each day is very important in that it sets the tone for all that follows. Breakfast-time is a good opportunity for setting a routine, but it also gives the patient choice, for instance whether to have cereal or not, or which cereal to have. The timetable must allow, wherever possible, for this sort of choice to take place.

In those centres where Conductive Education is solely practised the Conductors work shift hours, making it possible to develop a timetable that enables the patient to carry over all tasks that have been learnt in a practical manner (Fig. 5). For example, patients who have learnt to sit freely are given ample opportunity to practise this skill. The Conductor ensures that the patient performs to his best ability and in the correct way every time.

It should be obvious that the principle of continuity and transfer of skills is essential to help patients in a learning programme, although it may seem impossible for therapists to develop a closely-knit programme because of their own prescribed working timetable. Providing the timetable allows for learning experiences, however, some of the mechanics of management may be overcome. We have suggested

(p. 5) how the Conductor principle can be initiated. A different attitude and framework must be established which does not only rely on friendly co-operation between staff (the multi-disciplinary team) but also on forward planning, as in the inter-disciplinary team where a programme is constructed by all involved personnel, leading to specific goal attainment. Gradually all staff will inter-relate and be able to substitute for one another, producing a trans-disciplinary team. This in turn will hopefully develop into some staff being able to act as Conductors.

It may be useful for the reader to compare the sample timetable with patterns of activity that exist within their own establishment and to note in particular how much inactive time patients have, what opportunity there is for good walking, how often sitting position is corrected and whether functional activities enhance the patient's ability. From these observations the reader can devise his or her own appropriate timetable to give maximum learning facilitation to the patients.

Example of a timetable

Time	Activities	Staff
7–9 am	Getting up Washing—bath Dressing Breakfast	
9–9.30	Moving to day-room; supervised *good* walking	Shift 1
9.30–12 noon	Task-series in lying free sitting standing or walking	Two or three Conductors
12–12.30	Supervised *best* walk back to ward, or in day-room	
12.30–1.30	Lunch with Conductors	
1.30–2.30	Rest	Staff meeting of all Conductors
2.30–3 pm	*Good* walking to day-room or from rest place in day-room	
3–5 pm	Task-series at a table followed by functional activities relevant to task-series, etc *Best* walk to ward	Shift 2 Two or three Conductors
5–7 pm	Tea Free activities—reading, writing, etc Television Supper Preparation for bed Going to bed	

The code

As the Conductor develops and builds Task-series it becomes apparent that certain sequences of the code are frequently used and can therefore be condensed. These are denoted by the individual capital letters X,Y,Z and are explained as they occur during the task-series. As these three sequences are considered the most important in the development of functional skills, the Conductor and the patient must memorize the sequences in each of them.

The authors have developed this code to be used as a shorthand when carrying out and developing the task-series.

The code is constructed using combinations of letters of the alphabet to denote actions and numerals to denote position:

As Conductors become conversant with the task-series they can use the code as a shorthand. The intentions are denoted by letters and numerals, but there will be cases where there is no coding, in which case the intentions must be written in full.

a — I clasp my hands
a1 — I clasp my hands between my knees

Code

a   'I clasp my hands'

a1	between my knees
a2	on the table
a3	sidelying
a4	supine

b   'I stretch my elbows'
c   'I lift my arms up'

c1	clasped hands
c2	cl. hands ins. out
c3	L + R hand
c4	both hands
c5	basket

d   'I put my hands down'

d1	clasped hands
d2	cl. hands ins. out
d3	L + R hand
d4	both hands
d5	basket

X—a b c d = putting two hands on the table (see p. 28)
e   'I turn my clasped hands inside out'
f   'I part my hands'

f1	starting little finger
f2	starting index

Y—a b c d e f + m f1 = putting hands flat on the table (see p. 30)
g   'I put my palms on the table' (flat hands)
h   'Fingers straight'
i   'My hands are hanging down'
j   'I push my hands forward'

j1	clasped hands
j2	cl. hands inside out
j3	L + R hand
j4	both hands
j5	basket

Code

k	'I pull my hands towards me'	k1	clasped hands
		k2	cl. hands inside out
		k3	L + R hands
		k4	both hands
		k5	basket
l	'I support myself on my hands'	l2	clasped hands inside out
		l4	two flat hands
m	'I press my thumb-tips together'		
n	'I stand up'		
o	'I bend my elbows'	o1	standing
		o2	sitting at table—elbows fixed
p	'I sit down'		
q	'I put the back of my hand on the back of the table' (supination–outward rotation)		
		q1	clasped hands
		q2	L – R hands separate—straight elbows
		q3	L + R hands separate—bent elbows
		q4	both hands
		q5	basket
r	'Basket'	Index r2	
		Middle r3	
		Ring r4	
		Little r5	

Z *'Forming basket'* X Y + r2 r3 r4 r5 = Z (see p. 34)

st	Starting position		
s	'I put my foot flat on the floor'	s1	both feet flat on the floor
t	'I put my heel on my other knee'		
u	'I stretch my leg'		
v	'I take my foot to the side'	v1	straight leg
		v2	knee bent
w	'I put my foot back in the middle'	w1	straight leg
		w2	knee bent

PART
TWO
Task-series

28

Task-series sitting at a table
Sitting at the table teaches the patient:−
- to sit and lean forwards away from the back of the chair
- to use his arms to maintain his sitting position
- to use his good side for comparison
- to use visual feedback
- to use propioceptive feedback
- to observe others

Task I Learning to put two hands flat on the table.
Observation of patients

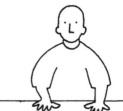

Task-series 1

Code: to use the code it is necessary to refer to the code (EC RK) on page 25

st: (starting position) Sitting at arm's length distance from the table. The table should be at normal desk height and the patients' feet flat on the floor. The patients should be well spaced and patients with similar problems close to one another.

Code	Rhythmical intention (ri)*	
i	My hands are hanging down	(1−5)
a1	I clasp my hands	(1−5)
b	I stretch my elbows	(1−5)
c1	I lift my arms up	(1−5)
d1	I put my hands down (on the table)	(1−5)
i	My hands are hanging down	(1−5)

* From now on Rhythmical Intention will be written as ri (p. 14)

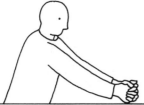 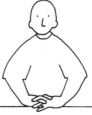

Task series 2		
Code		ri
st	as I.1	
i	My hands are hanging down	(1–5)
a1	I clasp my hands	(1–5)
b	I stretch my elbows	(1–5)
c1	I lift my arms up	(1–5)
d1	I put my hands down	(1–5)
j1	I push my hands forward	(1–5)
k1	I pull my hands towards me	(1–5)
e	I turn my hands inside out	(1–5)
b	I stretch my elbows	(1–5)
k2	I pull my hands towards me	(1–5)
i	My hands are hanging down	(1–5)

X* (bracket spanning a1, b, c1, d1)

X* For task-series sitting at a table X refers to clasped hands on the table and is made up of a, b, c, d performed in sequence. From now onwards X will constantly appear and readers should refer back to this page if in doubt of the sequence.

Task series 3		
Code		ri
st	as I.1	
i	My hands are hanging down	(1–5)
X		
e	I turn my hands inside out	(1–5)
j2	I push my hands forward	(1–5)
k2	I pull my hands towards me	(1–5)
m	I press my thumb tips together	(1–5)
n	I stand up	(1–5)
l	I support myself on my hands	(1–5)
m	I press my thumb tips together	(1–5)
b	I stretch my elbows	(1–5)
p	I sit down	(1–5)
i	My hands are hanging down	(1–5)

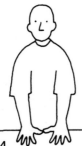

Task series 4

Code		ri
st	as I.1	
i	My hands are hanging down	(1–5)
a1	I clasp my hands	(1–5)
e	I turn my hands inside out	(1–5)
c2	I lift my arms up	(1–5)
d2	I put my hands on the table	(1–5)
b	I stretch my elbows	(1–5)
k2	I pull my hands towards me	(1–5)
m	I press my thumb tips together	(1–5)
j2	I push my hands forward	(1–5)
k2	I pull my hands towards me	(1–5)
n+b	I stand up and stretch my elbows	(1–5)
o	I bend my elbows	(1–5)
b	I stretch my elbows	(1–5)
p	I sit down	(1–5)
i	My hands are hanging down	(1–5)

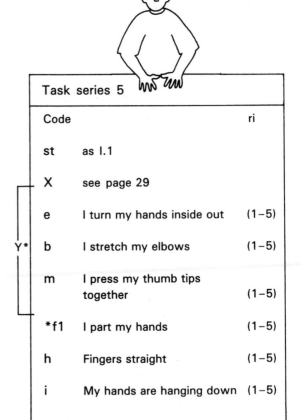

Task series 5

Code		ri
st	as I.1	
X	see page 29	
e	I turn my hands inside out	(1–5)
b	I stretch my elbows	(1–5)
m	I press my thumb tips together	(1–5)
*f1	I part my hands	(1–5)
h	Fingers straight	(1–5)
i	My hands are hanging down	(1–5)

Y*

Y* *From this point forward the sequences that make up Y will refer to flat separated hands on the table. Y is made up of X (a, b, c, d) plus e, b, m and f1. It is again understood that the patient will perform the complete sequence. From now onwards wherever Y appears readers should refer back to this page if in doubt of the sequence.*

*f1 I part my hands, starting with the little finger

Task II Learning to stand up and sit down at the table, stretching elbows, wrists and fingers.

Observation of patients

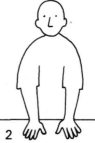

Task-series 1		
Code		ri
st	as Task I.1	
i	My hands are hanging down	(1–5)
a1	I clasp my hands	(1–5)
b	I stretch my elbows	(1–5)
c1	I lift my arms up	(1–5)
d1	I put my hands down	(1–5)
b	I stretch my elbows	(1–5)
e	I turn my clasped hands inside out	(1–5)
n	I stand up	(1–5)
l	I support myself on my hands	(1–5)
b	I stretch my elbows ⎤(×3)	(1–5)
o1	I bend my elbows ⎦	(1–5)
b	I stretch my elbows	(1–5)
p	I sit down	(1–5)
b	I stretch my elbows	(1–5)
m	I press my thumb tips together	(1–5)
f1	I part my hands	(1–5)
k4	I pull both my hands towards me	(1–5)
i	My hands are hanging down	(1–5)

Task-series 2		
Code		ri
st	As Task I.1.	
a2	I clasp my hands on the table	(1–5)
b	I stretch my elbows	(1–5)
e	I turn my clasped hands inside-out	(1–5)
b	I stretch my elbows	(1–5)
n	I stand up	(1–5)
l	I support myself on my hands	(1–5)
o1	I bend my elbows	(1–5)
b	I stretch my elbows	(1–5)
m	I press my thumb tips together	(1–5)
f1	I part my hands	(1–5)
b	I stretch my elbows	(1–5)
l	I support myself on my hands	(1–5)
o1	I bend my elbows	(1–5)
b	I stretch my elbows	(1–5)
p	I sit down	(1–5)
i	My hands are hanging down	(1–5)

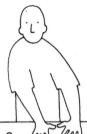

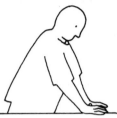

Task-series 3		
Code		ri
st	As Task I.1.	
X	see page 29	
e	I turn my clasped hands inside out	(1–5)
b	I stretch my elbows	(1–5)
k2	I pull my hands towards me	(1–5)
n	I stand up	(1–5)
l	I support myself on my hands	(1–5)
b	I stretch my elbows	(1–5)
m	I press my thumb tips together	(1–5)
	Move hands right – to middle, to left, to middle	
b	I stretch my elbows	(1–5)
p	I sit down	(1–5)
i	My hands are hanging down	(1–5)

Task-series 4		
Code		ri
st	As Task I.1.	
i	My hands are hanging down	(1–5)
X	see page 29	
b	I stretch my elbows	(1–5)
n	I stand up	(1–5)
e	I turn my clasped hands inside-out	(1–5)
j2	I push my hands forwards	(1–5)
k2	I pull my hands back	(1–5)
	Repeat j2 k2 3 times bending forward from the waist	
p	I sit down	(1–5)
i	My hands are hanging down	(1–5)

Task III Learning outward rotation of the arm and supination of the hand.
Observation of the patients

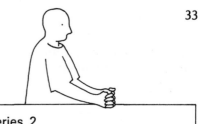

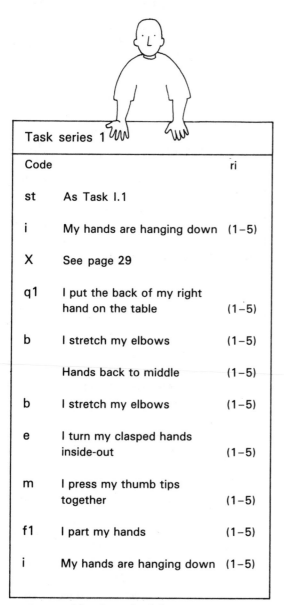

Task series 1		
Code		ri
st	As Task I.1	
i	My hands are hanging down	(1–5)
X	See page 29	
q1	I put the back of my right hand on the table	(1–5)
b	I stretch my elbows	(1–5)
	Hands back to middle	(1–5)
b	I stretch my elbows	(1–5)
e	I turn my clasped hands inside-out	(1–5)
m	I press my thumb tips together	(1–5)
f1	I part my hands	(1–5)
i	My hands are hanging down	(1–5)

repeat with q1 to the left

Task series 2		
Code		ri
st	As Task I.1	
Y	See page 30	
q2	I put the back of my right hand on to the table	(1–5)
b	I stretch my elbows	(1–5)
a2	I clasp my hands (on table)	(1–5)
b	I stretch my elbows	(1–5)
e	I turn my clasped hands inside out	(1–5)
m	I press my thumb tips together	(1–5)
f1	I part my hands	(1–5)
q2	I put the back of my left hand on the table	(1–5)
a2	I clasp my hands (in middle)	(1–5)
b	I stretch my elbows	(1–5)
e	I turn my clasped hands inside out	(1–5)
m	I press my thumb tips together	(1–5)
f1	I part my hands	(1–5)
b	I stretch my elbows	(1–5)
i	My hands are hanging down	(1–5)

Task IV Learning to form a basket.
Observation of patients

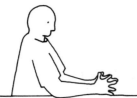

Task-series 1		
Code		ri
st	As Task I.1	
i	My hands are hanging down	(1–5)
Y	see page 30	
m	I press my thumb tips together	(1–5)
r2	I press the tips of my index fingers together	(1–5)
r3	I press the tips of my middle fingers together	(1–5)
r4	I press the tips of my ring fingers together	(1–5)
r5	I press the tips of my little fingers together	(1–5)
h	Fingers straight (and press)	(1–5)
i	My hands are hanging down	(1–5)

A basket Z is formed by performing the following sequences.*		
a	I clasp my hands	(1-5)
b	I stretch my elbows	(1-5)
c	I lift my arms up	(1-5)
d	I put my hands down	(1-5)
e	I turn my clasped hands inside out	(1-5)
b	I stretch my elbows	(1-5)
m	I press my thumb tips together	(1-5)
f1	I separate my hands	(1-5)
m	I press my thumb tips together	*1.*
r2	I press my index fingers together	*2.*
r3	I press my middle fingers together	*3.*
r4	I press my ring fingers together	*4.*
r5	I press my little fingers together	*5.*

* The sequences a, b, c, d, (X) + e, b, m, f1, (Y) + m, r2, r3, r4 and r5 collectively form a basket and are denoted by the letter Z. The reader will also note that the rhythm for the basket is 1. 2. 3. 4. 5. This gives a count for each finger, the underlying indicating the finger pressure. Wherever Z occurs in the text from now onwards readers should refer back to this page if in doubt of the sequences.

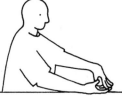

Task-series 2		
Code		ri
st	As Task I.1	
i	My hands are hanging down	(1–5)
Z	see page 34	
*q5	I turn the basket over to the right	(1–5)
	Back to the middle	(1–5)
q5	I turn the basket over to the left	(1–5)
	Back to the middle	(1–5)
b1	I stretch my elbows	(1–5)
m	I press my thumb tips together	(1–5)
f2	I part my hands, starting with the index	(1–5)
k5	I pull my hands towards me	(1–5)
i	My hands are hanging down	(1–5)

Task-series 3		
Code		ri
st	As Task I.1	
i	My hands are hanging down	(1–5)
Z	see page 34	
b	I stretch my elbows	(1–5)
m	I press my thumb tips together	1.
	I press all my finger tips together	2. 3.
c5	I lift the basket up	(1–5)
d5	I put the basket down	(1–5)
		(× 3)
i	My hands are hanging down	(1–5)

In the code q is I put the back of my hand on the table (pronation and supination). When in the basket position patients find it easier if the word basket is used. I turn the basket over.

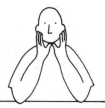

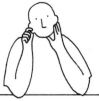

Task-series 4		
Code		ri
st	As Task I.1	
i	My hands are hanging down	(1–5)
Z	see page 34	
o2	I bend my elbows (fix elbows on the table)	(1–5) (×3)
	Basket on the table	(1–5)
o2	I bend my elbows	(1–5)
m	I press my thumb tips together	(1–5)
f2	I part my hands and hold my chin (palms on face, thumbs under chin)	(1–5)
h	Fingers straight	(1–5)
i	My hands are hanging down	(1–5)

Task-series 5		
Code		ri
st	As Task-series 4 up until f2	
	Bend head to left and hold left ear between finger and thumb	(1–5)
	Back to middle holding ear	(1–5)
	Bend head to right and hold right ear between finger and thumb	(1–5)
	Back to middle holding both ears	(1–5)

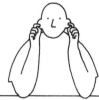

Task-series 6		
Code		ri
st	As Task I.1	
i	My hands are hanging down	(1–5)
Z	see page 34	
o2	I bend my elbows and hold my ears	(1–5)

Task V Learning to bend and stretch
individual fingers.
Observation of patients

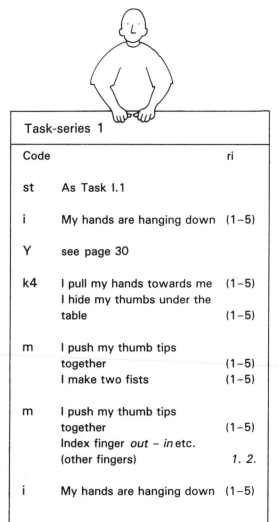

Task-series 1		
Code		ri
st	As Task I.1	
i	My hands are hanging down	(1–5)
Y	see page 30	
k4	I pull my hands towards me	(1–5)
	I hide my thumbs under the table	(1–5)
m	I push my thumb tips together	(1–5)
	I make two fists	(1–5)
m	I push my thumb tips together	(1–5)
	Index finger *out – in* etc. (other fingers)	*1. 2.*
i	My hands are hanging down	(1–5)

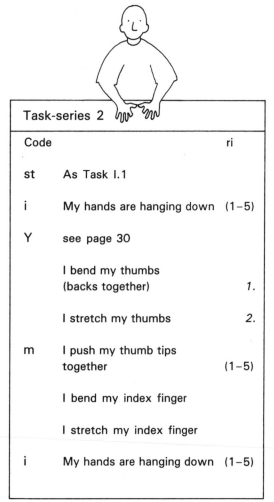

Task-series 2		
Code		ri
st	As Task I.1	
i	My hands are hanging down	(1–5)
Y	see page 30	
	I bend my thumbs (backs together)	*1.*
	I stretch my thumbs	*2.*
m	I push my thumb tips together	(1–5)
	I bend my index finger	
	I stretch my index finger	
i	My hands are hanging down	(1–5)

If possible repeat m to include all fingers

Task VI Learning to raise the arms up high.
Observation of patients

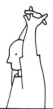

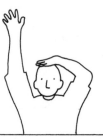

Task-series 1		
Code		ri
st	As Task I.1	
i	My hands are hanging down	(1–5)
b	I stretch my elbows	(1–5)
a2	I clasp my hands	(1–5)
e	I turn my clasped hands inside out	(1–5)
c2	I lift my arms up (above head)	(1–5)
m	I press my thumb tips together	(1–5)
f1	I part my hands	1. 2. 3. 4. 5.
h	Fingers straight	(1–5)
a	I clasp my hands in the air above my head	(1–5)
d1	I put my hands down	(1–5)

Task-series 2		
Code		ri
st	As Task I.1	
Y	see page 30	
b	I stretch my elbows	(1–5)
a2	I clasp my hands	(1–5)
c1	I lift my arms up	(1–5)
e	I turn my clasped hands inside out	(1–5)
m	I press my thumb tips together	(1–5)
f1	I part my hands 1. 2. 3. 4. 5. R hand remains straight in the air or rests on the top of a ladderback while the L hand touches the top of the head, or the back of the neck, or the opposite shoulder, elbow or wrist. I touch my . . .	(1–5)
b	I stretch my elbow	(1–5)
a	I clasp my hands	(1–5)
d1	I put my hands down	(1–5)

Task VII Learning to place palmar side
of the wrist on the forehead.
Observation of patients

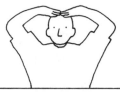

Task-series 1		
Code		ri
st	As Task I.1	
i	My hands are hanging down	(1–5)
X	see page 29	
e	I turn my clasped hands inside out	(1–5)
b	I stretch my elbows	(1–5)
c2	I lift my arms up	(1–5)
b	I stretch my elbows	(1-5)
	I put my palms on my head	(1–5)
	I put my R wrist on my forehead	(1–5)
	Palms on my head	(1–5)
	I put my L wrist on my forehead	(1–5)
	Palms on my head	(1–5)
a	I clasp my hands	(1–5)
e	I turn my clasped hands inside out	(1–5)
c2	I lift my arms up	(1–5)
b	I stretch my elbows	(1–5)
d2	I put my hands down	(1–5)
i	My hands are hanging down	(1–5)

Functional tasks relevant to the task-series are introduced as early as possible to motivate the patients and to give them concrete goals to work towards. The Conductor must select these tasks according to the patients' ability and interests as well as enabling the patients to perform these tasks in their free time.

The following photographs are examples of functional tasks (fig. 6. 7. 8.)

In the task-series sitting at a table the patient will have progressed from two-handed activities (hands clasped) through to fine finger movements. The choice of functional tasks is endless but performance is most successful when the Conductor has prepared the tasks herself and directly related these to the group, the individuals and the task-series.

40

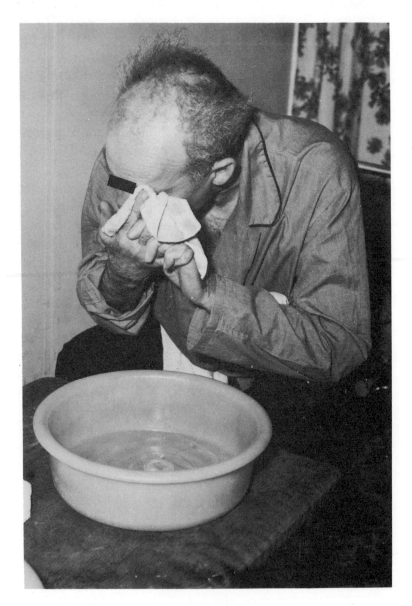

Fig. 6 Functional tasks: washing—two-handed activity (clasped hands)

41

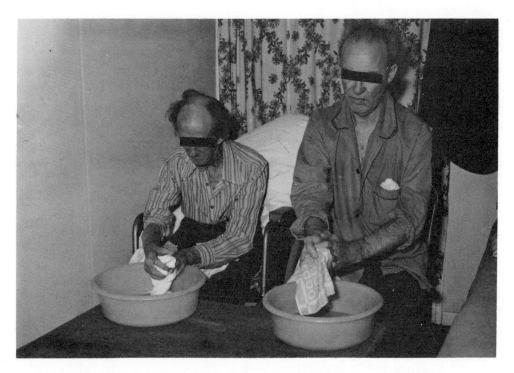

Fig. 7 Functional tasks: washing—two-handed activity (hands apart)

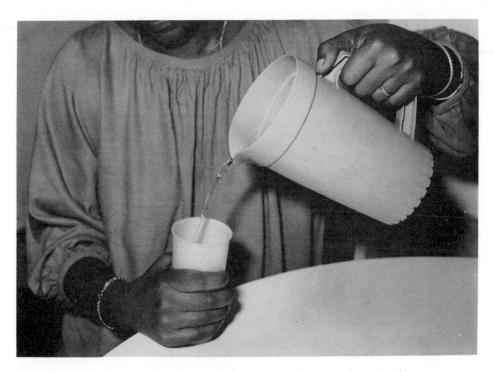

Fig. 8 Functional tasks: pouring—two-handed activity (one hand fixed, one hand moving)

Task-series in lying

In the first stages of his illness the patient works in the lying position on the bed or plinth.

From the very first moment active stretching of the elbow, wrist and fingers is attempted. These movements are active/passive, the unaffected side assisting the affected side. The patient should soon reach the stage where by stretching his fingers he can hold a stick placed in his hand. If he cannot stretch his fingers he will learn to hang his arm down and loosen his hand with the help of gravity and ri.

Task-series in lying are practised on a slatted plinth. The slats can be used for grasping and the height of the plinth facilitates sitting down, lying down and standing up as used in all activities linked to getting in and out of bed.

Getting up and down from the floor is best linked with the free-sitting task-series so that the patients can learn to get down from the chair and use the chair when getting up again.

On the whole task-series in the lying position are easier than those in sitting and standing as gravity is not counteracting the movement of the arm. The trunk is well supported and the supine position also facilitates extension of the arm.

On the other hand, the patients may find the pre-walking task-series which combine arm, trunk and leg movements more complicated than the task-series in sitting where visual feed-back is a facilitator.

Task I Learning to lift and lower clasped hands.
Observation of patients

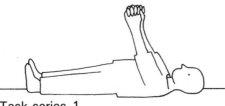

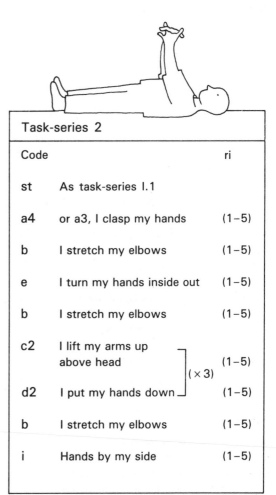

Task-series 1		
Code		ri
st	As in the sitting task-series the patients must learn to find the correct starting position with or without ri. Arms at the side, elbows straight, palms down. Head in the middle. Legs straight, feet dorsiflexed, legs externally rotated. 'If finding this starting position were easy, the patients would not need our help'. (Petö)	
	When necessary the patients loosen the arm and hand hanging the arm down from the plinth. Gravity and ri are the facilitators	
a4	or a3 I clasp my hands	(1–5)
b	I stretch my elbows	(1–5)
c1	I lift my arms up above head	(1–5)
b	I stretch my elbows	(×3) (1–5)
d1	I put my hands down	(1–5)

Task-series 2		
Code		ri
st	As task-series I.1	
a4	or a3, I clasp my hands	(1–5)
b	I stretch my elbows	(1–5)
e	I turn my hands inside out	(1–5)
b	I stretch my elbows	(1–5)
c2	I lift my arms up above head	(1–5)
d2	I put my hands down	(×3) (1–5)
b	I stretch my elbows	(1–5)
i	Hands by my side	(1–5)

Task II Learning to lift and lower parted hands.

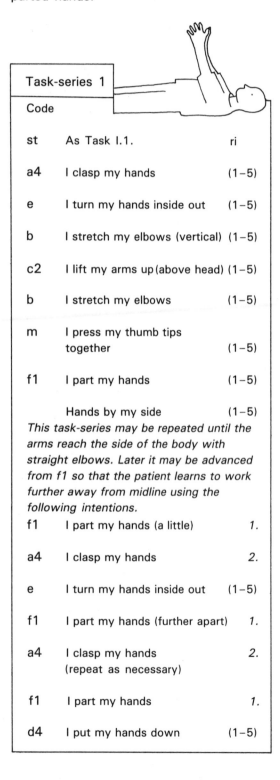

Task-series 1

Code		
st	As Task I.1.	ri
a4	I clasp my hands	(1–5)
e	I turn my hands inside out	(1–5)
b	I stretch my elbows (vertical)	(1–5)
c2	I lift my arms up (above head)	(1–5)
b	I stretch my elbows	(1–5)
m	I press my thumb tips together	(1–5)
f1	I part my hands	(1–5)
	Hands by my side	(1–5)

This task-series may be repeated until the arms reach the side of the body with straight elbows. Later it may be advanced from f1 so that the patient learns to work further away from midline using the following intentions.

f1	I part my hands (a little)	1.
a4	I clasp my hands	2.
e	I turn my hands inside out	(1–5)
f1	I part my hands (further apart)	1.
a4	I clasp my hands (repeat as necessary)	2.
f1	I part my hands	1.
d4	I put my hands down	(1–5)

Task-series 2.

Code		ri
st	As Task I.1.	
a4	I clasp my hands	(1–5)
e	I turn my hands inside out	(1–5)
b	I stretch my elbows	(1–5)
c2	I lift my arms up (above head)	(1–5)
m	I press my thumb tips together	(1–5)
f1	I part my hands	1.
d4	I bring my hands down (vertical position)	2.
c4	I lift my arms up (above head)	3.
a4	I clasp my hands (above head)	4.
e	I turn my hands inside out	(1–5)
m	I press my thumb tips together	(1–5)
fl	I part my hands	1.
d4	I bring my hands down (lower than vertical)	2.
c4	I lift my arms up (above head)	3.
a4	I clasp my hands (above head)	4.
e	I turn my hands inside out	(1–5)
m	I press my thumb tips together	(1–5)
repeat f1, d4, c4, d4 as above		
	Hands by my side	5.

Repeat as possible and when necessary

Task III Learning to put one hand on the opposite shoulder, elbow or wrist. Observation of patients

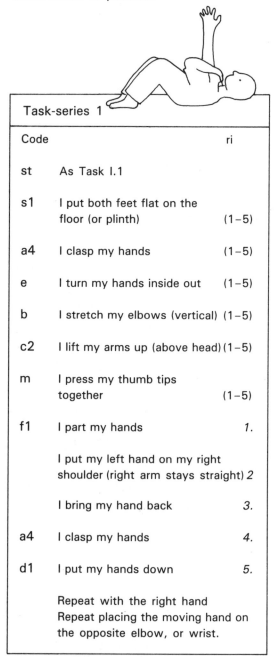

Task-series 1		
Code		ri
st	As Task I.1	
s1	I put both feet flat on the floor (or plinth)	(1–5)
a4	I clasp my hands	(1–5)
e	I turn my hands inside out	(1–5)
b	I stretch my elbows (vertical)	(1–5)
c2	I lift my arms up (above head)	(1–5)
m	I press my thumb tips together	(1–5)
f1	I part my hands	*1.*
	I put my left hand on my right shoulder (right arm stays straight)	*2*
	I bring my hand back	*3.*
a4	I clasp my hands	*4.*
d1	I put my hands down	*5.*
	Repeat with the right hand Repeat placing the moving hand on the opposite elbow, or wrist.	

The Intention
'I put both feet flat on the floor' is used deliberately and demonstrates how language may be used to describe more than one action, in this instance flexion of both hip and knees.

Task IV Learning to make a basket. Observation of patients

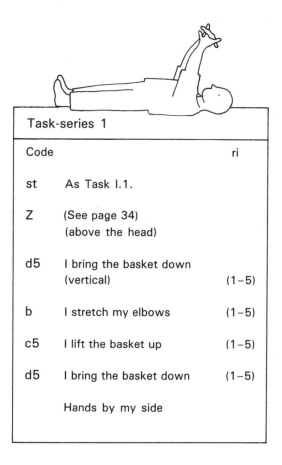

Task-series 1		
Code		ri
st	As Task I.1.	
Z	(See page 34) (above the head)	
d5	I bring the basket down (vertical)	(1–5)
b	I stretch my elbows	(1–5)
c5	I lift the basket up	(1–5)
d5	I bring the basket down	(1–5)
	Hands by my side	

Task V Learning to place palmar side of the wrist on the forehead.

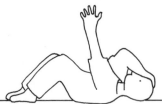

Task-series 1		
Code		ri
st	As Task I.1	
Z	(See page 34) (above the head)	
f2	I part my hands	(1–2)
	I put my left hand on my head	*1.*
	Left hand back	*2.*
a4	I clasp my hands	(1–5)
Z	(See page 34)	
f2	I part my hands	*1.*
	I put my right hand on my head	*2.*
	Right hand back	*3.*
a4	I clasp my hands	*4.*
d1	I put my hands down	*5.*
	Hands by my side	

Repeat, but instead of putting the moving hand on the head, put it on the opposite shoulder or hold the nose or opposite ear.

Task VI Working with one or two sticks

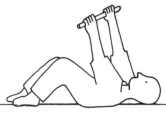

All these tasks are done using ri
1.   Grasp a stick in both hands. Lift the stick vertically, above the head and down. Elbows must be straight, wrists extended and the patients must follow the stick with their eyes. Repeat with thin stick, held by index and thumbs.
2.   Hold a smaller stick in either hand. Lift together vertically, above the head and down. Watch L or R stick successively. Place the L then the R stick on the ear.
3.   Hold one stick in both hands. Lift the stick up vertically and above the head. Let go with L hand. Move the R arm holding the stick down to the plinth, and back up again. Grasp the stick. Ditto with the other hand. Stick down.
4.   Hold stick vertically in both hands. Lift the stick a bit 1. Turn the stick, L, R and back in the middle 2.3.4. Lift again 1., turn 2.3.4. Repeat all the way up and down again.

Task VII Learning to put feet flat on the floor

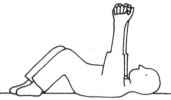

Task-series 1		
Code		ri
st	As Task I.1	
a4	I clasp my hands	(1–5)
b	I stretch my elbows	(1–5)
	I turn on my left side	(1–5)
	I bring my top foot to my knee	(1–5)
	I turn on my back	(1–5)
s	I put my foot flat on the floor	(1–5)
u	I stretch my leg slowly	(1–5)
	Repeat for other leg	
a4	I clasp my hands	(1–5)
s1	I put both feet flat on the floor	(1–5)

Task VIII Learning to turn onto the side

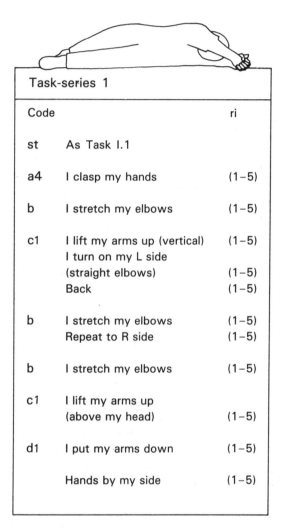

Task-series 1		
Code		ri
st	As Task I.1	
a4	I clasp my hands	(1–5)
b	I stretch my elbows	(1–5)
c1	I lift my arms up (vertical)	(1–5)
	I turn on my L side (straight elbows)	(1–5)
	Back	(1–5)
b	I stretch my elbows	(1–5)
	Repeat to R side	(1–5)
b	I stretch my elbows	(1–5)
c1	I lift my arms up (above my head)	(1–5)
d1	I put my arms down	(1–5)
	Hands by my side	(1–5)

Task IX Learning to place supinated hands under the buttocks.
Observation of patients

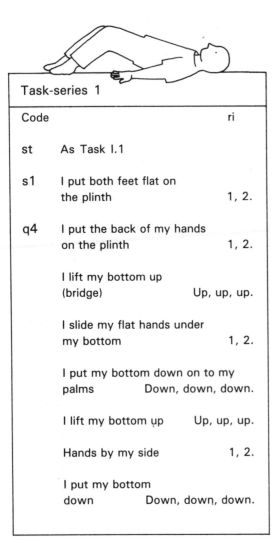

Task-series 1

Code		ri
st	As Task I.1	
s1	I put both feet flat on the plinth	1, 2.
q4	I put the back of my hands on the plinth	1, 2.
	I lift my bottom up (bridge)	Up, up, up.
	I slide my flat hands under my bottom	1, 2.
	I put my bottom down on to my palms	Down, down, down.
	I lift my bottom up	Up, up, up.
	Hands by my side	1, 2.
	I put my bottom down	Down, down, down.

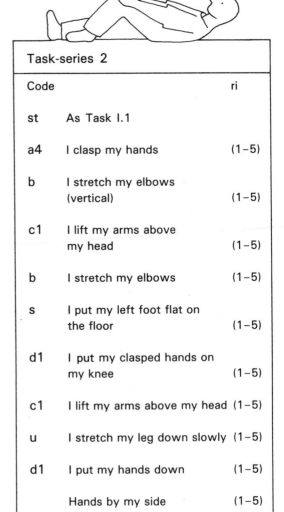

Task-series 2

Code		ri
st	As Task I.1	
a4	I clasp my hands	(1–5)
b	I stretch my elbows (vertical)	(1–5)
c1	I lift my arms above my head	(1–5)
b	I stretch my elbows	(1–5)
s	I put my left foot flat on the floor	(1–5)
d1	I put my clasped hands on my knee	(1–5)
c1	I lift my arms above my head	(1–5)
u	I stretch my leg down slowly	(1–5)
d1	I put my hands down	(1–5)
	Hands by my side	(1–5)
	Repeat with the other leg	

Task X Learning to place the heel of the foot on the other knee

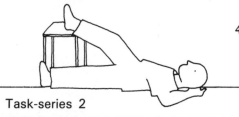

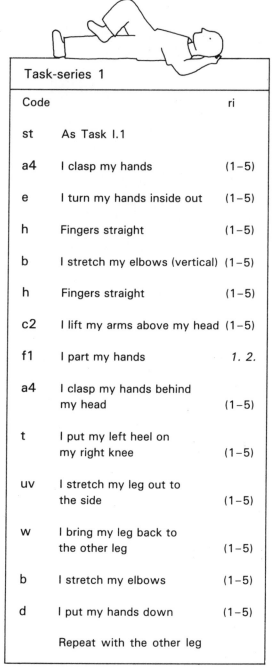

Task-series 1

Code		ri
st	As Task I.1	
a4	I clasp my hands	(1–5)
e	I turn my hands inside out	(1–5)
h	Fingers straight	(1–5)
b	I stretch my elbows (vertical)	(1–5)
h	Fingers straight	(1–5)
c2	I lift my arms above my head	(1–5)
f1	I part my hands	1. 2.
a4	I clasp my hands behind my head	(1–5)
t	I put my left heel on my right knee	(1–5)
uv	I stretch my leg out to the side	(1–5)
w	I bring my leg back to the other leg	(1–5)
b	I stretch my elbows	(1–5)
d	I put my hands down	(1–5)
	Repeat with the other leg	

This task-series breaks up the flexor pattern of the arm and the extensor pattern of the leg.

Task-series 2

As task-series 1, but if the patient cannot lift his leg to place the heel on the knee, a chair or stool may be put under his foot so he can move the foot from the chair to the knee.

Task-series 3

As task-series 1, but instead of stretching the leg to the side the patient moves the heel slowly from the knee along the shin of the other leg until he reaches the foot, counting slowly to 5.

Task-series 4

As 1, 2, and 3 adding dorsiflexion of the foot when the heel is placed on the knee *(up-down)* keeping the dorsiflexion when stretching the leg.

The task-series in lying are a direct preparation for walking. Patients learn to move one leg whilst the other remains stationary and also learn to fix the hands (preventing associated reactions) by clasping hands (fig. 9), holding a stick or holding the slats on the plinth (fig. 10). Arm movements are preparatory to all functional tasks (fig 11a & b). Being able to lift the arms enables the patient to sit up which involves simultaneous stretching of the arms and flexion of the hips. Rolling from side to side enables the patient to take weight through the elbows prior to long sitting (see fig. 12).

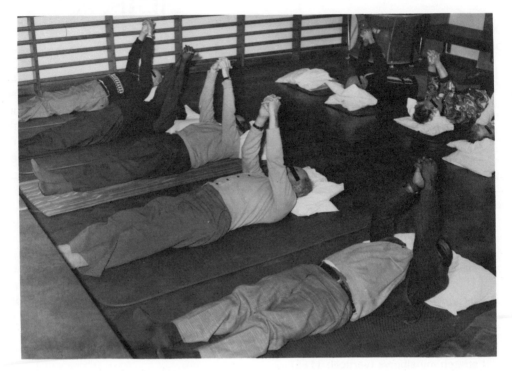

Fig. 9 Clasping hands and stretching elbows

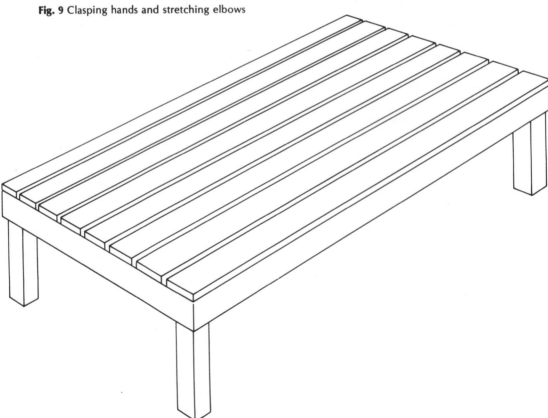

Fig. 10 Slatted plinth

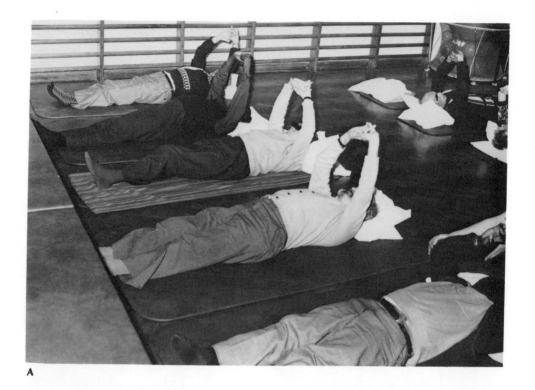

A

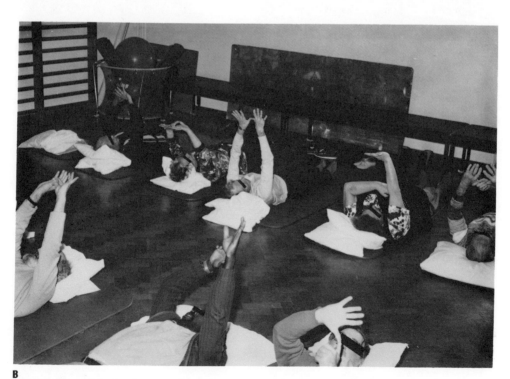

B

Fig. 11 Parting of the hands A. Hands inside out B. Thumbs pushed together

52

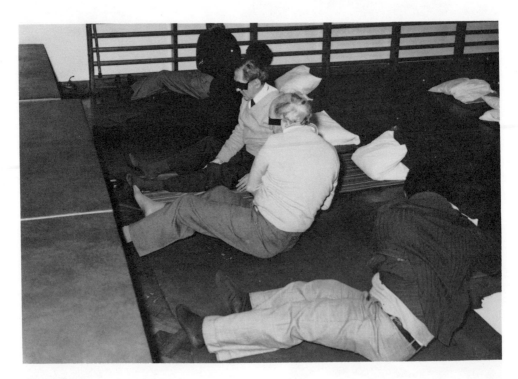

Fig. 12 Coming up into sitting

Task-series in free-sitting

Free-sitting improves sitting and
develops sitting balance.
Free-sitting assists unsupported
movement of the hemiplegic arm.
Free-sitting is a preparation for
standing up, standing and walking.
The aid used in the free-sitting
task-series is the ladderback chair
(fig. 13).

Task I Learning to work with the
hemiplegic arm.
Observation of patients

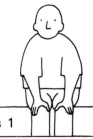

Task-series 1		
Code		ri
st	Knees and feet slightly apart, feet flat. The hands are on the knees, thumbs inside the knee. The head is in midline. This position is first found with or without the aid of ri. Very soon the patients will know the position and will find it themselves and check it themselves. In this way they learn their position in space and how to experience the idea of the midline.	
i	My hands are hanging down	(1–5)
a1	I clasp my hands	(1–5)
b	I stretch my elbows	(1–5)
c1	I lift my arms up (above head)	(1–5)
b	I stretch my elbows	(1–5)
d1	I bring my hands down (on knees)	(1–5)
i	My hands are hanging down	(1–5)

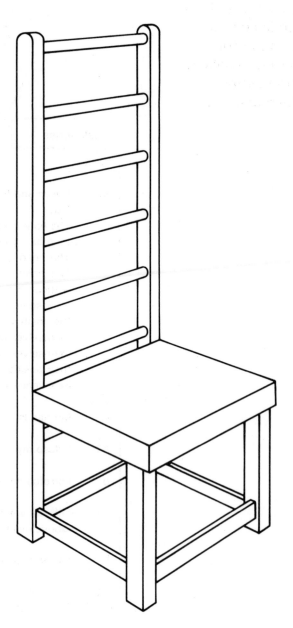

Fig. 13 Ladder-back chair

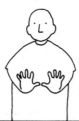

Task series 2		
Code		ri
st	As task-series I.1	
i	My hands are hanging down	(1–5)
*X	(See page 29)	
c1	I lift my hands up half way	(1–5)
e	I turn my hands inside out	(1–5)
b	I stretch my elbows	(1–5)
m	I press my thumb tips together	(1–5)
f2	I part my hands	1.
d4	I put my hands down on knees	2.
i	My hands are hanging down	(1–5)

In task series in free sitting X refers to clasped hands on the knees but the sequences are the same as on page 29.

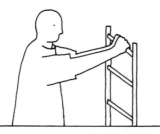

Task-series 3

Code		ri
st	As Task I.1. with a ladder back chair in front	
i	My hands are hanging down	(1–5)
X	See page 29	
c1	I lift my arms up (above head)	(1–5)
e	I turn my hands inside out	(1–5)
b	I stretch my elbows	(1–5)
m	I press my thumb tips together	(1–5)
f1	I part my hands	1.
	I place my hands on the top rung (with a straight elbow)	2.
a	I clasp my hands (eye level)	(1–5)
b	I stretch my elbows	(1–5)
e	I turn my hands inside out	(1–5)
m	I press my thumb tips together	(1–5)
fl	I part my hands	1.
	I place my hands on the ladder (half way up)	2.
i	My hands are hanging down	(1–5)

This task-series is repeated at varying heights with some patients attempting all heights, other perhaps only one level. A further progression would be:—

fl	I part my hands	1
	I hold my straight arms	2
	I place my hands on the rung	3

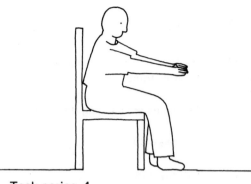

Task II Learning to stand up from free-sitting.
Observation of patients

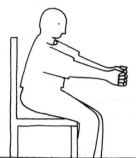

Task-series 4		
Code		ri
st	As Task I.1	
*Y	See page 30 (halfway up)	
d4	I bring my hands down (on knees)	1
c4	I lift my arms up	2
d4	I bring my hands down	3
Y	See page 30 (above head)	
d4	I bring my hands down	1
c4	I lift my arms up	2
d4	etc. etc. at varying heights, using ladderback when necessary. Some patients may be able to lower the arm freely but not lift it, others may need the use of *m* as a facilitation.	3
i	My hands are hanging down (1–5)	

In task-series in free sitting Y refers to unsupported hands with straight elbows, wrists and fingers.

Task-series 1		
Code		ri
st	As Task I.1.	
i	My hands are hanging down	(1–5)
a1	I clasp my hands	(1–5)
b	I stretch my elbows	(1–5)
	I bend forward	(1–5)
b	I stretch my elbows	(1–5)
	I lift my bottom up	(1–5)
	I stretch my knees	(1–5)
n	I stand up	(1–5)
p	I sit down slowly	(1–5)

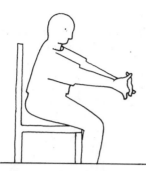

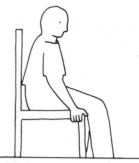

Task-series 2		
Code		ri
st	As Task I.1.	
i	My hands are hanging down	(1–5)
al	I clasp my hands	(1–5)
b	I stretch my elbows	(1–5)
e	I turn my hands inside out	(1–5)
b	I stretch my elbows	(1–5)
	I lift my bottom up	(1–5)
n	I stand up	(1–5)
p	I sit down	(1–5)
i	My hands are hanging down	(1–5)

Task-series 3		
Code		ri
st	Sitting grasping the seat of the chair, with the thumbs on top	
	I bend forward	(1–5)
b	I straighten my elbows	(1–5)
	I press my feet into the ground	(1–5)
	I lift my bottom up	(1–5)
n	I stand up	(1–5)
p	I sit down	(1–5)

58

Task III Learning to stand up with a
ladderback chair.
Observation of patients

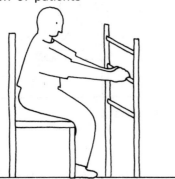

Task-series 1		
Code		ri
st	As Task I.1. with a ladderback chair in front of the patient	
i	My hands are hanging down	(1–5)
Y	(See page 30) at eye level	
	I grasp the chair	(1–5)
	I push the chair forward	(1–5)
b	I stretch my elbows	(1–5)
	I lift my bottom up	(1–5)
n	I stand up	(1–5)
p	I sit down	(1–5)

Task IV Learning to part the legs and turn.
Observation of patients

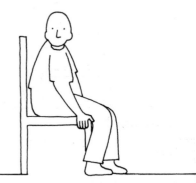

Task-series 1		
Code		ri
st	As Task I.1.	
v2	I put my left foot to the left and turn	1.
w2	Back to the middle	2.
	Repeat with the right foot and turn (The hands can stay on the knees and act as a facilitation or grasp the seat of the chair as Task II No. 3 Page 57) This task can be developed so that the foot is placed round the corner of the chair.	
v2	I put my left foot to the left (round the corner)	1.
	I put my right foot by my left	2.
w2	Right foot back to the middle	1.
w2	Left foot back to the middle	2.
	Repeat to the other side	

Task V Learning to lift and abduct the leg.
Observation of patients

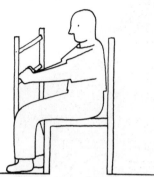

Task-series 1		
Code		ri
st	As Task I.1	
	A ladderback chair is in front of the patients with the back of the chair facing the patients	
i	My hands are hanging down	(1–5)
Y	(See page 30) I grasp the chair	(1–5)
v2	I put my left foot on the left side of the chair (flat)	1.
	I put my left knee on the frame of the chair	2.
	I slide my foot up	3.
	I slide my foot down	4.
w2	I put my foot back in the middle	5.

repeat with other leg

Task VI Learning to lift the leg with flexed
knee and dorsi-flexed foot.
Observation of patients

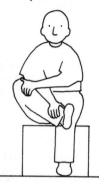

Task-series 1		
Code		ri
st	As Task I.1	
i	My hands are hanging down	(1–5)
	I grasp the chair with thumb on top	(1–5)
	I put my right heel on my left knee	1.
	I grasp my ankle with my right hand	2.
	I put my left hand on my knee	3.
	I push my knee down	4.
	I put my foot on the floor	5.

Free-sitting task-series develop good sitting, sitting balance and the ability to stand up (fig 13, 14, 15, 17).
Functional tasks are putting on shoes, socks, and stockings which are best relearnt in free-sitting (fig 16).

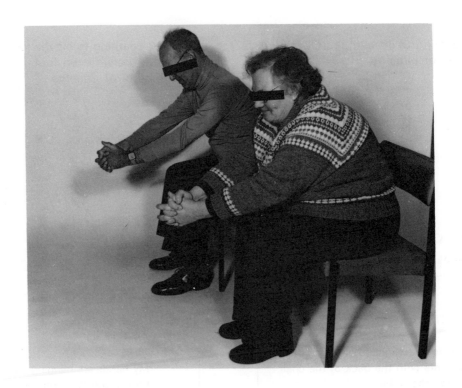

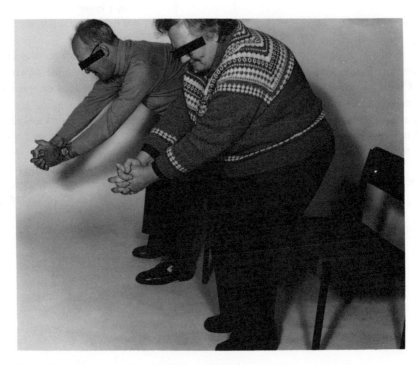

Fig. 14 Learning to stand up with clasped hands

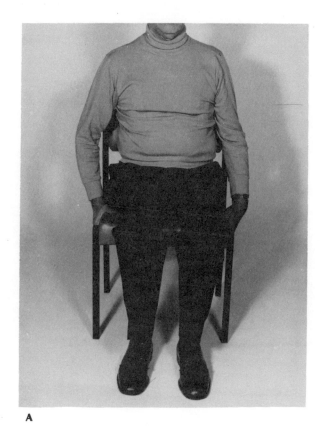

A

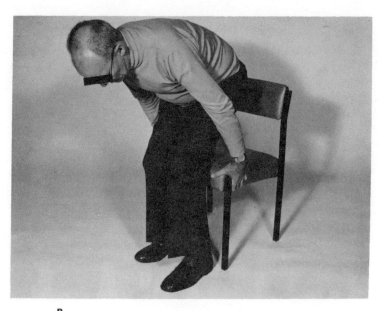

B
Fig. 15 A. Learning to stand up B. Pushing up from the chair

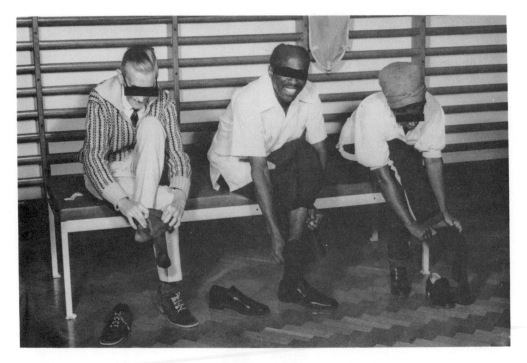

Fig. 16 Putting on socks

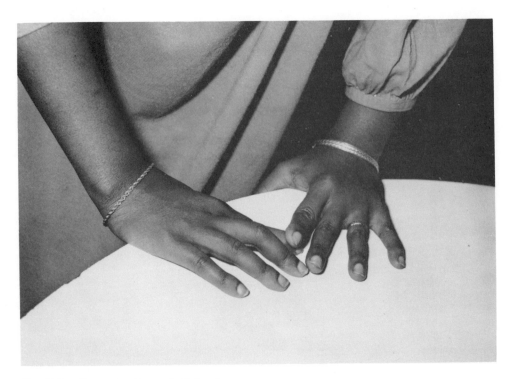

Fig. 17 Standing supporting on both hands

Task-series in standing

The purpose of task series in standing is to prepare the patient for walking. The patient has learnt to stand up through task series in sitting at a table — Task II 1, 2, 3, 4, Page 31 task series in free sitting — Task II 1, 2, 3, Page 56 Task III 1. Page 58

Task I Learning to weightbear on the hemiplegic leg.
Observation of patients

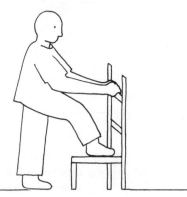

Task-series 1	
Code	ri
st	Standing in front of a ladderback chair with the seat facing the patient. The patient grasps the ladder, the arms in 90° elevation, (having used Y. see page 30).
	I put my weight on my right leg (1–5)
	I put my left foot on the chair *1.*
	I bend my knee and elbows *2.*
b	I stretch my elbows *3.*
	I put my foot down slowly (1–5)
	Repeat with the other leg

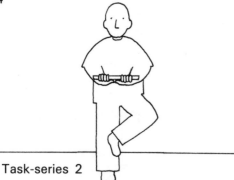

Task-series 2	
Code	ri

st Depending on the patients ability
the starting position will be:
Standing — grasping a ladderback
chair with 2 hands
— between 2 chairs
grasping with
2 hands
— between 2 chairs
grasping with
1 hand
— with one chair at
the side grasping
with the affected
hand
— holding a stick in
both hands (elbows
extended)
or
— holding a stick in the
affected hand

I put my weight through
my right leg   (1–5)

t I put my left heel on
my right knee   *1.*

I put my heel back on
the floor   *2, 3, 4, 5.*

(The foot is everted and
dorsiflexed)

Task-series 3	
Code	ri

st As Task I.2

I put my weight on my
right leg   (1–5)

I put my left heel forward   *1.*

I put my left foot back   *2.*

Repeat with the other leg

See also task-series X in lying page 49

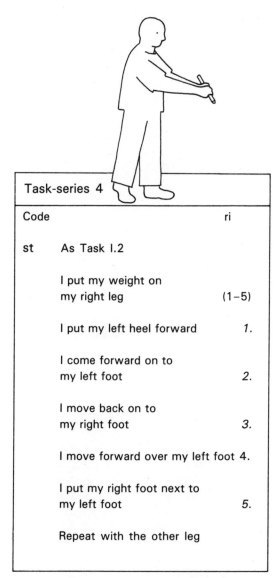

Task-series 4

Code		ri
st	As Task I.2	
	I put my weight on my right leg	(1–5)
	I put my left heel forward	*1.*
	I come forward on to my left foot	*2.*
	I move back on to my right foot	*3.*
	I move forward over my left foot	*4.*
	I put my right foot next to my left foot	*5.*
	Repeat with the other leg	

The patient should learn to rock forward and backward weightbearing over a straight leg

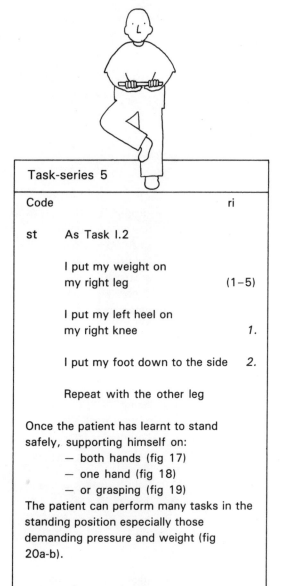

Task-series 5

Code		ri
st	As Task I.2	
	I put my weight on my right leg	(1–5)
	I put my left heel on my right knee	*1.*
	I put my foot down to the side	*2.*
	Repeat with the other leg	

Once the patient has learnt to stand safely, supporting himself on:
— both hands (fig 17)
— one hand (fig 18)
— or grasping (fig 19)
The patient can perform many tasks in the standing position especially those demanding pressure and weight (fig 20a-b).

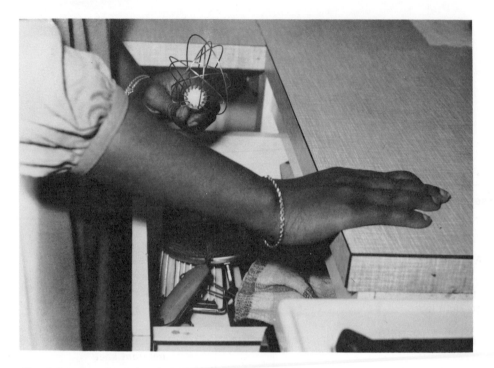

Fig. 18 Standing supporting on one hand

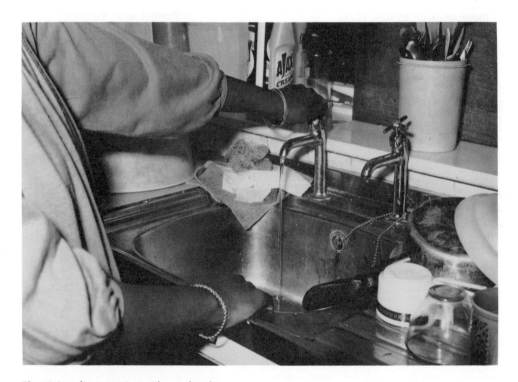

Fig. 19 Standing grasping with one hand

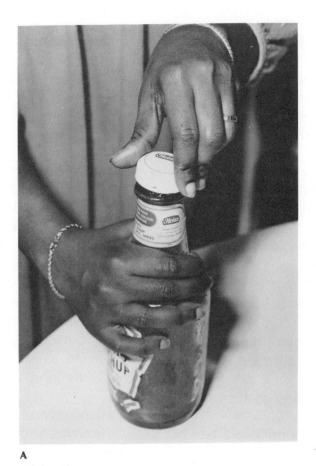

A

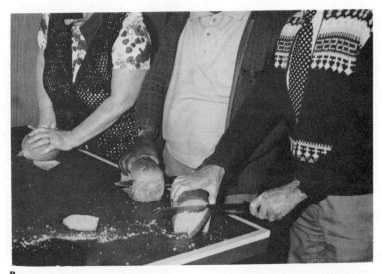

B
Fig. 20 Standing using grasp, pressure and weight A. Opening a bottle
B. Cutting bread

Task-series in walking

Observation of patients
The hemiplegic patient has difficulty with walking because:—
a. He cannot take his body-weight on the affected leg when taking a step with the unaffected leg — and
b. When stepping forward with the affected leg he circumducts the leg with a stiff knee and plantarflexed, inverted foot, the toes scraping the floor.

The patients have been prepared for walking in many different positions.

see: Task-series sitting at a table Task II 1, 2, 3, 4. Task-series in lying VII 1, IX 1, 2, X 1, 2, 3, 4. Task-series in free sitting II 1, 2, 3. Task-series in standing.

The patient should have learnt:
1. To shift his weight from one leg to the other.
2. To weightbear on either leg.
3. To bend one leg while keeping the other leg straight.
4. To control himself in midline.
5. To move his legs and control the bending of the affected arm.

The Conductor knows what the patient has learnt and how the patient performs. With this knowledge and rhythmical intention, walking is practised. This may be by:—
- pushing a ladderback chair with two hands
- between 2 rows of ladderbacks
- grasping a stick in both hands
- grasping a stick in the affected hand (to avoid associated reactions)
- walking with hands on the buttocks, or one buttock (to assist hip extension)
- walking with a pole.

Patients who have minimal walking difficulties should practise synchronized armswing. This is extremely difficult even for those patients who have developed hand function. The automatic armswing has to be re-learnt and if practised during work sessions must be kept up throughout the rest of the day. The rhythmical intention used in walking should vary and will depend upon:
- the patient's ability
- the walking speed of the patient and the support currently being used by the patient to facilitate walking.

Some examples of the variations
may be:

● — push-step, step, stand
● — weight on one leg   *1.*
   — step with the other leg   *2.*
● — heel to knee   *1.*
   — step   *2.*

During the day the patient will
practise his 'best walking'
according to his individual ability.
This will include going to the toilet,
to meals and other activities when
he will be *supervised* by the
Conductor. Apart from the 'best
walking' the patient should use his
'next best walking' or 'traffic
walking' when *unsupervised.*
These will at a later stage be
discarded for 'best walking'. The
photographs shown illustrate the
preparation of walking (figs 21, a,
b, c & d).

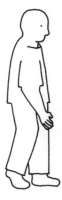
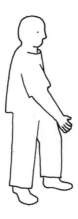
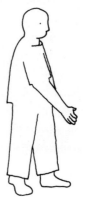

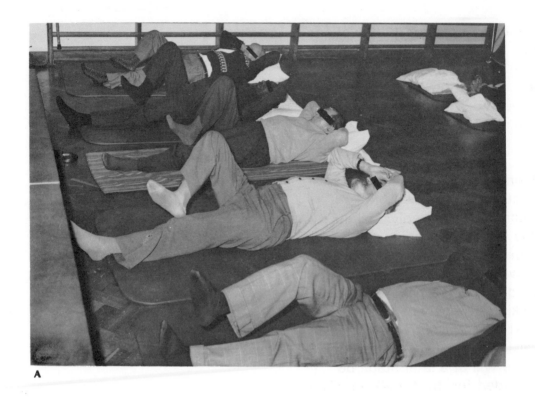

A

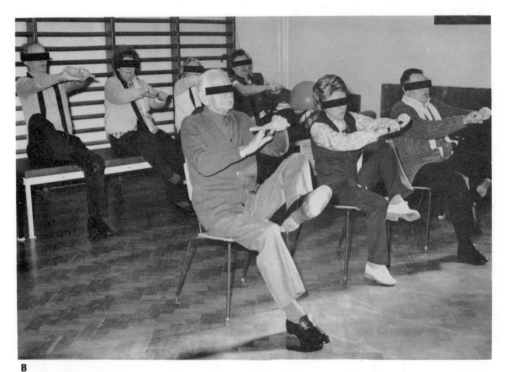

B

Fig. 21 Examples of preparation for walking A. In lying B. In sitting

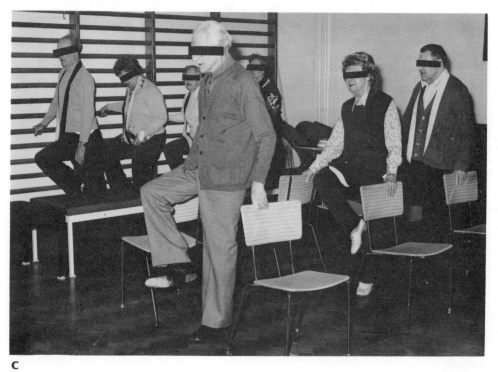

C

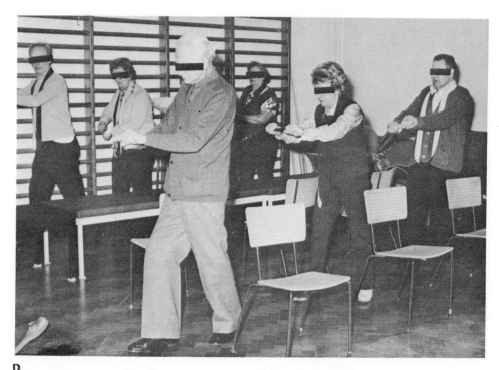

D

Fig. 21 Preparation for walking C. Between two chairs D. Unsupported

REFERENCES

Annett J 1969 Feedback on human behaviour. Penguin
  Books, Harmondsworth
Bernstein N A 1967 The co-ordination of movements.
  Pergamon Press, Oxford
Betchenov 1866 Reflexes of the brain. St Petersburg, p 3
Dickinson A 1981 Conditioning and associative learning.
  Medical Bulletin 37(2)
Elliot J, Connolly K 1973 The growth of competence.
  Academic Press, London
Frolov Y P 1937 Pavlov and his school. Kegan Paul,
  Trench, Trubner, London
Heal L W 1972 An analysis of the evaluation and follow-up
  data from the Institute for Conductive Education of
  Motor Disabled in Budapest, Hungary. University of
  Wisconsin Press, Madison, Wisconsin
Hilgard E R, Atkinson R L, Atkinson R C 1953 Introduction
  to psychology, 7th edn. Harcourt Brace Jovanovich,
  New York
Institute for Conductive Education of the Motor Disabled
  1975 Scientific studies on Conductive Education.
  Conductor's College, Budapest
Luria A R 1961 The role of speech in the regulation of
  normal and abnormal behaviour. Pergamon Press,
  Oxford
Luria A R 1973 The working brain. Penguin Books,
  Harmondsworth
Luria A R, Yudovich F 1968 Speech and the development
  of mental processes in the child. Staples Press,
  St Albans
Sherrington C S 1934 The brain and its mechanism.
  Cambridge University Press
Vygotsky L S 1962 Thought and language. M.I.T. Press,
  Cambridge, Massachusetts